EAT, THINK AND BE SLENDER

Eat, Think and Be Slender
New and Revised

LEONID KOTKIN, M.D.

with FRED KERNER

AN AUTHORS GUILD BACKINPRINT.COM EDITION

Eat, Think and Be Slender

AN AUTHORS GUILD BACKINPRINT.COM EDITION

Published by iUniverse.com, Inc.

For information address:
iUniverse.com, Inc.
620 North 48th Street, Suite 201
Lincoln, NE 68504-3467
www.iuniverse.com

Originally published by Hawthorn

ISBN: 0-595-00394-X

Printed in the United States of America

For JEAN, JON, GARTH and BETH

To protect the identity of individuals involved in the case studies included in this book, the names, occupations and other circumstances have been altered. The essential clinical material is factual and true.

How many men are kept busy to humor a single belly!

—Seneca: EPISTULAE AD LUCILIUM

Contents

Contents

Contents

The Solution

Preface

THE PROBLEM OF OBESITY is one which confronts millions of persons. Each and every overweight man and woman has at one time or other attempted to do something about this serious problem. Few have succeeded.

Most have failed for two simple reasons: they did not understand why they had grown obese and they did not seek the help of a physician in combating this disease. Therein lies the very basic principle of weight reduction. Each of the reasons is contingent upon the other if a cure is to be effected.

If the obese person does not understand the cause of his illness, the physician cannot help him. If the obese person does not go to the physician for help, he cannot learn to understand the basis of his illness.

To this end *Eat, Think and Be Slender* was written. I do not believe in starving the dieter. In fact, on the contrary, I allow the dieting patient to eat as much as he wants, the only limitation being that the foods forbidden by the diet may not be touched at all during the dieting.

The obese person should not feel that he is not going to get enough to eat. But before he goes on the diet, the patient must be made to think about the root of the problem. He must be made to understand why he has grown overweight, why he must lose weight, why success is necessary in the diet regime, and how success can be achieved. Understanding then becomes equally as important as dieting in the treatment of the obese person.

So I admonish the obese: eat, think and be slender.

While this book was written principally for the layman, it has another important purpose. Many doctors are called upon to help patients lose excess weight, but too often the doctor's efforts are in vain because of psychological blindness on the part of the patient. A great many patients have a psychological block against seeing themselves as they really are. The patient looks in the mirror and sees himself a slim, handsome man-about-the-campus as, perhaps, he was years before. But worse still, he refuses to see his obesity is caused purely by overeating.

This book, then, will give the busy practitioner a better opportunity to help obese patients. The average physician has too little time to devote several hours to each patient who comes to him with the problem of overweight. Yet it sometimes takes many hours of discussion to root out the direct cause of the patient's obesity and then to help the patient understand this cause and effect in his particular case.

For these busy doctors, *Eat, Think and Be Slender* will provide a handbook to help their patients acquire the insight necessary to combat the problem. Their patients having a readily available means of obtaining the necessary insight, the busy physicians will be able to start right in on the essential business of curing the disease.

For their help in the preparation of this volume, I would like to acknowledge the aid of and offer my sincerest thanks to the United States Public Health Service, the W. B. Saunders Company, Dr. Norman Jolliffe, Dr. Hilde Bruch, Marguerite Clark of *Newsweek,* and Jean Kotkin.

I wish to express my appreciation to Fred Kerner for his help in the preparation of this book.

14   Leonid Kotkin, M.D.

THE PROBLEM

Understanding Obesity ─────────────────

O, that this too too solid flesh would melt. . .

Shakespeare: HAMLET

A NUMBER OF NEW PATIENTS come to my office daily, worrying about a new "inflation" sweeping the land—the physical inflation of inches added to their waistlines.

This has brought to my attention the stark reality that, despite all that has been written about obesity, too few persons have been able to overcome the problem.

Yet there is no reason why, if you are overweight, you should not be able to lose weight and then hold the advantage thus gained in the later years of your life.

You have undoubtedly discovered by hard experience that losing weight is not accomplished overnight. But your past failures do not mean that it cannot be done. It can—and you can do it.

The solution lies principally within yourself.

Persons who were overweight for years have taken off all their excess poundage and have admitted that the results were almost unbelievable. The road to reducing is more easily traveled than you imagine if you are willing to complete the journey and accept the fact that the hazards encountered en route are surmountable.

17

At the outset you must take two simple steps: Go to a doctor. Allow him to help you understand why you are obese.

Overweight is a "disease" for which the most important medicine needed is understanding. Understanding—that is, insight to the problem responsible for the excess weight—is essential to achieve a cure.

The treatment of obesity is divided into five parts—I call it the "Quinary Rule." The Quinary Rule comprises PSYCHOTHERAPY (to help you understand why you are fat); HIGH-PROTEIN DIET (so that you can lose weight while *continuing to eat as much of the permissible foods as you want*); HUNGER-CURBING MEDICATION (so that you can help restrain your hunger); VITAMIN SUPPLEMENTS (to maintain your health level); and WEIGHT-WATCHING (so that you can eventually maintain your normal weight without difficulty).

The benefits of this treatment are not only immediate. They have long-range effects as well.

The best evidence to show that weight control pays has been compiled by the Metropolitan Life Insurance Company. They have made a study of persons who were obese and succeeded in losing sufficient weight so that they could qualify for insurance. This study showed that the death rate after weight reduction was substantially less than that for all obese persons studied.

There is no *abracadabra* which can be said over a fat body to have it turn thin. There is no gadget which can be employed to achieve the effect. No amount of only counting calories on little pocket charts, nor any set of diets alone will do the trick.

Your doctor will help you first to understand why you are obese. Then he will set about helping you lose weight. He will prescribe hunger-curbing medication; he will prescribe additional vitamins if needed; he will carefully plan a diet for you; he will help bolster your morale when you may feel that there is a possibility of failure.

Your doctor can calculate the amount of nutritional fuel your body needs with amazing accuracy. He will consider the amount of exertion you are subjected to, the loss of your body heat due to atmosphere, and the amount of internal work your body does. This may sound fantastic to you, but it is not so. This computation is made in units you know so well from the publicity they have received in the popular press—calories.

Actually a calorie is only a unit of heat. It is used in computing the heat of the body's energy needs just as British Thermal Units —or BTUs—are used in computing a building's heat requirements. Technically a calorie is the amount of heat required to raise the temperature of one thousand grams (more than $2\frac{1}{5}$ pounds) of water one degree centigrade ($1\frac{4}{5}$ degrees Fahrenheit).

So that you may have an idea of how food can be computed in calories in figuring out the body's needs, consider that one single gram (about $\frac{1}{33}$ of an ounce) of protein or carbohydrate produces four calories. That means that such an infinitesimal quantity of food could raise the temperature of more than two pounds of water more than seven degrees Fahrenheit. One gram of fat produces nine calories.

The diet your doctor prescribes is planned with particular care for your own specific case. There are many fine points to be considered in making a diet. Your own vitamin and mineral needs must be taken into account, for if your diet fails to supply essential dietary needs (and many ready-made diets may), it can be exceedingly dangerous.

When you read of the results which have been achieved by this method of weight reduction, you may be inclined to think that the claims are a little extravagant. Actually they are all cases selected from my files as a cross-section so that among them you may perhaps recognize your own particular troubles.

This will offer you, then, a mirror by which you can see inside yourself so that you may acquire the all-important understanding of obesity.

Obesity is not a glandular disease, nor is it a metabolic disease.

19

That is to say there is no gland in the body capable of manufacturing *fat out of air and water,* nor will one person's normal digestive processes manufacture more fat out of the same amount of food than another person's.

Simply, obesity is the product of an emotional disturbance. Being overweight is a definite expression on the part of the individual. It is either a suit of armor to crudely cloak many anxieties, or an excuse by which the individual avoids mature responsibilities.

Bluntly, obese persons form a definite group of immature patients in exactly the same way as do alcoholics, drug addicts, anxiety neurotics, and character psychoneurotics.

Just as the theoretical concept of "normal" does not exist in reality, so one cannot dogmatically assert that all overweight persons are completely emotionally immature. As a trait, however, obesity points unfailingly to a neurotic personality.

The best definition of an obese individual is one who, if left to his own devices in regulating his food intake, will compulsively exhibit an abnormal accumulation of excess fat. That is to say, persons whose neuroses express themselves in their growing fatter are compelled psychologically to gain weight as a cover-up for some fear, some failing, some lack. One might label them *obesity-compulsives.*

These persons envy their neighbors who have normal waist-lines. They fondly hope, and eagerly search, for a magic recipe that will allow them to satisfy the compulsive cravings they experience for food and yet retain, or attain, the physical appearance of their favorite Hollywood star.

These persons are fair game for quacks and miracle-men, who abound. They avidly digest the advertisements in newspapers and magazines, and on television and radio, which sell "sure-cure treatments" such as vitamin supplements, bulk laxatives, exercise parlors and contraptions designed to remove unsightly fat from all unfavorable places.

The books written about obesity could fill a "Five-Foot Shelf." New ones appear almost constantly. Some contend that as long as a fat person has the correct information regarding the caloric value of all foods, and uses a series of charts and menus, he will be able to reform his evil ways and become sylphlike. Others treat the subject lightly, probably with the idea that you can laugh fat away by reading the witty remarks, limericks and gags (with appropriate cartoons) concerning the trials and tribulations of a "fatty" during a diet regime.

None of the books written to date, however, has taken into consideration that the reader—be he an obese person, or someone interested in the problem of obesity for other reasons—is intelligent enough to truly understand why people become obese and to understand the processes, both emotional and organic, which contribute to overweight.

This book has been written with no idea of spoon-feeding the reader. Herein you will find no tear-off-on-the-dotted-line charts to keep with you for restaurant meals, no algebra (nor even arithmetic) to calculate in calories, no "open sesame" to the treasure trove of svelte slimness.

There is only one formula—and there is no magic about it. It is what I call the P and Q formula: To watch your Ps you must mind your Qs. That is to say, to watch your *poundage*, you must mind your *Quinary Rule*. Turn to the beginning of this chapter and read it again.

The first and last of these five rules are the ones in which you play the greatest part. First you must understand why *you* are fat. Then your doctor can utilize rules two, three and four. When you have gained your goal, you have to set out to be a weight-watcher lest those prodigal pounds return.

So watch your Ps and mind your Qs.

The Fortress of Fat _____

Not for renewal, but for eating's sake,
They stuff their bellies.

Edmund Vance Cook: BOOK OF THE EXTENUATIONS

MANY PEOPLE ARE INSECURE and feel unable to cope with the onslaughts of a "cruel and demanding world."

A great percentage of these insecure people are obese. While there are many reasons—unconscious ones—for attaining a large girth, one of the most frequently found is insecurity.

Who is to determine whether you are going to be secure or insecure? You yourself!

And, if you allow yourself the doubtful attribute of insecurity, you may well become one of the obese. One of the easiest ways of shirking the responsibilities of living is by hiding. And one of the most common ways of hiding—as going into seclusion on a desert island is virtually an impossibility—is by building a "suit of armor" and climbing into it.

This suit of armor acts as a fortress to protect the insecure and the hypersensitive. It is a fortress of fat. There is little doubt that the person who becomes grossly obese is really building a fort around himself wherein he will feel safer as he goes about his daily life.

A lecturer in history at an eastern university was one of my earliest obesity patients. After "running away" within herself by building the protective coat of fattiness, she finally ran away physically and came to New York to start anew.

This young woman comes from a well-established family. She had acquired a great deal of respect among her colleagues as a teacher. Had you met her when she first came to New York, you would have classified her immediately as a good-natured fat girl. She was always jolly, always laughing. She was everyone's "pal" and would have gladly given the dress off her back to help any of her friends.

Of her jollity, she once said, however, "I've got to be jolly. I'm too big to run and too fat to fight."

She was so well insulated by fat that no one of her friends —or her family for that matter—knew her. Her fortress of fat was impregnable. All anyone knew of her was the surface, which, aside from a potentially pretty face, actually was quite unattractive.

Within this "vile castle" lived a beautiful princess and she, as in tales of old, was waiting for her Prince Charming to come to rescue her. Her dream prince undoubtedly was much like her favorite Hollywood star, though she was intelligent enough to have disdained such an idea consciously.

After lengthy discussions, she admitted, "I see where I really was running away from the real world with its many demands, its disappointments and its discipline.

"I must have been living in a dream world—though I didn't realize it."

Well, the Ugly Duckling legend won't come true other than in a dream world. A kiss from Prince Charming won't awaken the sleeping princess. Yet the beautiful lady can be released from her imprisonment in the tower of obesity, and this one was. She followed treatment carefully and successfully lost forty-three pounds in five months.

Another young woman employed by a research foundation was a similar case. Under her layers of fat she was a tangle of taut nerves.

"I have to be good-natured and obliging all the time to people," she said during an early interview, "otherwise my nerves will get the better of me and I'll say something that I'll be sorry for.

"And that's the easiest way I know of losing the good will, love and admiration of the friends I now have."

So great was the insecurity of this research worker, and so deep-rooted, that she would not even show temper upon being abused by persons in friendship's name.

The specter of loneliness haunted her, and it was of her own making. It need never have been so and it was finally disposed of.

There was no need for her to have become trapped in the vicious circle of eating. Yet boredom, frustration and unhappiness led her down the fatal path of obesity. To cloak this unhappiness, she ate and ate and ate—and succeeded admirably in building layers and layers of fat into an unbreachable defense. When she succeeded in losing fifty-one pounds in about five months, she came out of her shell like a butterfly from a cocoon.

I recall yet another young lady. She was, and is still, a pleasant person. When she first came for treatment she was—on the surface —calm and good-natured. Her façade was one of jollity.

The very capable secretary to a successful member of the bar, her devotion and loyalty to her employer is well known by all in the legal profession. For that matter, work she did with her employer in helping the underprivileged brought her headline fame in many newspapers and magazines.

She is a woman of average height and, at the time, weighed 196 pounds, when she should have been about sixty pounds lighter.

"Every bit of my clothing has to be made for me," she told me, "because I cannot dress as befits my position and buy my clothes ready-made. Actually, to maintain the wardrobe I need takes a huge portion of what would be considered a very good salary."

Then came an old tale of woe.

"You know, Doctor, I hardly eat anything at all and yet there isn't a thing I can do to lose weight. I've tried all sorts of diets and they haven't worked. I guess it must be a glandular condition!

"My sister, who's only a little more than a year younger than I, eats as much as a horse and yet she doesn't put on an ounce. And every morsel I eat seems to turn into fat."

After she was oriented, this young secretary was willing to begin a proper regime of dieting. With her coming to understand the causes of her obesity, came the desire to accomplish something for herself—outside of her work—instead of remaining the insecure devoted slave to others.

I got a great deal of pleasure watching the *real self* emerge from the fatty shell. As she became more attractive, upon melting inches of the fortress away, conversations such as these occurred: "For the first time that I can remember, I actually told my boss that he was wrong the other day when he vented his anger on me for something his wife had done to him . . ."

And: "The nerve of her [*a friend*] even suggesting such a thing. Why she doesn't realize just how good a friend I am to her —and I told her so in no uncertain terms . . ."

She was acquiring the security she needed so that she could avoid being stepped on. She unconsciously allowed her temper to show itself when anger was warranted by unjust treatment.

Her employer, who is extremely dependent on her efficiency, came to regard her personal qualities with more respect when he discovered that she could no longer be treated as just a piece of office equipment.

She, on the other hand, became more tolerant of some friends who had become noticeably catty. She now realized that these girls were watching a new and formidable rival emerge from the shell of what had been an unattractive woman.

25

"You'd be surprised at the number of attempts that have been made to discourage me," she told me one day after we discovered that she had peeled off many telltale pounds.

"I've been ridiculed as being vain; and so often, when I go visiting friends, I've been served, or offered, the most tempting —but fattening—dishes and delicacies.

"Worst of all are the stories I've been told about the dangers of losing weight. Why, just the other day two good friends pointed out a story in the newspapers about an actor who died after dieting.

"Of course, the papers carried a report the next day that an incurable disease had been responsible."

These stories, I pointed out, often are used to hide the existence of such diseases as cancer. Persons who die of incurable diseases are often said to have died of other causes.

Once the underlying motives of all this frontal attack on her by her friends was understood, the patient acquired a reinforced determination to finish the job. There were, of course, periods of temporary backsliding. That is to be expected and will be discussed later in this book. Despite weeks where her weight went up instead of down, she attained her goal in six and a half months.

Having shed her fortress of fat, she is no longer the good-natured, jolly fat girl. But she has gained stature in the eyes of all who know her. She has been able to do this because she allowed herself to understand the reasons for her tendency to overeat.

She discarded the grandmothers' tales of harm in dieting, the quack rules and regulations of how to lose weight. She had enough faith in herself and courage to continue so that when we reached the point in the reducing regime where a temporary halt in the process was inevitable, she did not become discouraged.

Her approach to the situation was as ideal as could be found under the circumstances. Where previously she had been pitied and used by others, she now was respected and truly liked. She has outgrown many of her former friends, but she no longer needs that type of companionship. She has supplemented these persons with many new friends whom she has met through her work, something which would not have been possible a year previously.

This is not the end of the story, however.

Despite the wonderful success with this patient, there still is not completeness in the treatment. As I pointed out a few sentences back, everything was "as ideal as could be ... under the circumstances."

This patient could never attain true emotional understanding of her difficulties. She did have enough intellectual understanding to realize that her obesity was merely a cloak which shielded her from reality. But the mechanism—the very basic reason—behind this case was never unearthed because the patient would not consent to undergo psychoanalysis. She was satisfied with the results achieved and was willing to remain a *weight-watcher* to hold her poundage at an ideal level rather than get to the root cause of the obesity and turn it up to light so that, through emotional understanding, she would never again encounter the drive to put on weight.

She is no different from any of thousands of obese people in remaining a *weight-watcher*. While it is desirable for them to attain emotional understanding of their problems, this is not quite practicable for all cases.

The energies of the psychiatrist, analyst and psychotherapist are directed to the so-called major problems involving major psychoses, neuroses, anxiety states, hysterias, alcoholism and psychopathic personalities. These are often more dramatic and pressing problems than what I term *obesity-compulsion*.

Even if it were possible to explore the deep psychopathology in every case of obesity, the lack of sufficient trained personnel and the great expense to the patient for such highly trained technicians would make it prohibitive for many.

However, it is possible to deal with the problem from a practical point of view.

It is essential that all overweight persons be made to realize that their obesity is self-inflicted through unconscious mechanisms. All quackery in this field must be exposed so that many thousands of hopeful, but deluded, persons are not disillusioned and give up this important struggle.

Physicians must devote themselves more to this problem instead of treating it in an offhand manner. In spite of the knowledge obtained from so many clinical studies, some physicians still behave as though there is something "unclean" in treating a case of obesity.

While knowledge and technique are essential in helping the patient, the prime requisite is the patient's understanding of his problem. Without this there is not sufficient drive to get the treatment under way, and under these circumstances no weight reduction regime can succeed.

Too many books have been written on what to eat and what not to eat. Knowledge of food is important—but it is certainly not enough. It is doubtful whether one person in a hundred could ultimately succeed in removing fat permanently by knowing just what to eat and what to avoid.

In my experience, I have yet to meet a patient who did not know, as well as I, which foods are fattening and which are not. But this knowledge is only a minor facet in the treatment—and it best comes into play only after understanding is achieved.

In many cases, the realization alone that fat is a fortress and acts as a cloak to mask the *true you* is sufficient to trigger the determination to rid oneself of this suit of armor. Such persons can diet with little supervision provided they follow the rules of good nutrition involving abundant proteins, vegetables and vitamin supplements. Other cases will need the supervision of an understanding and sympathetic physician. There will be cases whose obesity is merely one of many neurotic traits. These cases frequently require more than intellectual understanding.

Such persons' deep-seated neuroses will throw up many blocks. They will be unable to give up the oral pleasures temporarily, yet it is only temporarily that they have to be subdued.

These persons require the attention of an expert technician in emotional problems. This is time-consuming and expensive. The dynamics of immaturity are not uncovered in a short time.

This fortress of fat is not the only expression of a personality in difficulties. There are many forms of "organ language." The entire field of psychosomatic medicine is full of them. Skilled actors, who are wonderful observers, have utilized a complete repertory of postures and gestures which convey many meanings not expressed by words.

Many of our slang expressions in common usage have created symptoms, such as a "pain in the neck," "my aching back," and "I'm fed up to here." Most pains in the neck, backaches and lumps in the throat complained about to doctors are protests against a life situation.

The individual living in a fortress of fat is saying to the world: "You can't reach me, you can't touch me; I'm safe here."

Is It Glandular?

The eye is bigger than the belly.

George Herbert: JACULA PRUDENTUM

PEOPLE ARE OBESE because they overeat!

Most overweight persons try to explain why they are fat. Many say their obesity is due to their glands. Some are quite specific. For instance, a stockbroker calmly announced on his first visit to my office, "I have an underactive thyroid gland!"

This man—who is a person of far greater than average intelligence—and all the other patients who have diagnosed their own problem don't half realize what they are saying. If they did they would not make such rash statements. First, they assume that there is some mysterious gland in the body which is capable of manufacturing fat out of air and water. This would be a wondrous thing indeed, but, unfortunately, science has failed to uncover such a gland in any member of the animal kingdom.

What is so-called glandular obesity? It is actually an unusual circumstance—and an unfortunate one—which causes excesses of fat to be deposited about the body in a peculiar fashion. But these "glandularly obese" persons still must overeat, or eat the wrong foods, in order to build up these deposits of fat.

30

Fat persons suffering from a glandular disturbance are treated no differently than other patients suffering from obesity—with one exception: cases of myxedema; that is, thyroid deficiency. Myxedema is relatively rare. Yet many overweight persons will seek to shift the blame away from themselves for their condition. They will almost invariably complain loudly to doctor and friends: "Oh, if it weren't for my underactive thyroid, I'd be as slim as you!"

They have picked up a ready-made excuse from some magazine article or newspaper item and have adopted it to shift the blame away from themselves. Rather than cutting down on the volume of their food intake, or checking to see if the foods they eat daily are good for them, these "excuse-seekers" would sooner overeat and complain. After all, with an excuse they believe, what more could they ask.

Time and again—and I am sure that this is an occurrence which happens in almost every doctor's office—I have had intelligent people offer this self-diagnosis of their condition.

In the past few months alone, a dress designer, an industrial engineer, a judge, and a high school teacher have offered this same bit of "help" to me. The shocking thing about hearing this excuse from such people is that I would expect them to think twice before deciding that this was what caused their trouble.

In each case I have patiently explained that if they had been suffering from an underactive thyroid the chances were one in a million that they would be anywhere near the heights they had reached in their respective professions. Certainly we know well enough that our social structure is such that only a person of above average intelligence can reach the higher strata of success in such specialized forms of livelihood.

The judge who came to me had gone even further than just saying he was suffering from an underactive thyroid. He had, with characteristic interest, taken the trouble to determine the medical term for the disease. Obviously he had not done any more research, because once he knew that obesity could be a symptom of myxedema, he was satisfied to latch on to it as his trouble.

Our meeting, at my office late one afternoon after court had been adjourned, ran something like this:

"Doctor, I've been gaining weight steadily for the past number of years and have been unable to do anything about it. Now I've discovered that I'm suffering from myxedema. Is there anything that can be done to help me?"

I imagine the expression on my face bothered the learned jurist. Before I had a chance to answer him, he went on: "I've heard of the success you had in my friend's case, so when I found out what my trouble was, I felt you could help me. I guess it's impossible, then?"

Now I had to cut in unless he imagined his initial visit—and the whole treatment—a failure before we had even started. I smiled at him.

"Now look here, Judge," I said. "It seems to me that as a man on the bench you would check a little deeper into a 'precedent.' After all, just because the end result is the same it surely doesn't mean that the entire case is the same.

"You wouldn't assume that because Mr. A was sentenced to five years' imprisonment that he had committed the identical crime as Mr. B who drew the same sentence.

"And yet, that is almost exactly what you are doing in your own case. Because thyroid underactivity will help cause obesity, you are willing to think that your excessive weight is also caused by myxedema. And, while I'm on the subject, I'm surprised to see that though you did research to find the medical name for the disease, you didn't bother to go on and delve into some of the other symptoms of this 'impossible thing' you are suffering from.

"First of all, a thyroid deficiency has an immediate effect on the intelligence capacity. Anyone with the mental capacity to reach your position in society could hardly be suffering from such a lack.

"Secondly, such persons are sluggish in everything they do. They react slowly to every stimulus. Walking along the street any doctor could—aside from the physical characteristics—pick out a myxedema case. You'll find such persons getting tangled up in ordinary sidewalk traffic; they'll find themselves crossing against red lights, because they didn't see them until they were half-way out in the street; they'll react slowly to any excitement around them.

"And thirdly, physically they are almost of a type. Textbooks always say that thyroid deficients look as though they come from the same family no matter what their origin. It is much like Mongoloid idiocy. The fattiness of such a person is a watery looseness that is equally deposited all around the body."

The jurist was smiling, recognizing the joke he had perpetrated at his own expense. In many ways it *was* funny. Here was a man whose intelligence, trigger-quick mind and keen perception had made him one of the most respected members of the legal profession, placing himself voluntarily in a class with a cretin.

Children who are born with thyroid deficiencies are labeled as cretins—and it is a step on the intelligence-scale only once removed from a Mongolian idiot. Such children can rarely develop normally. Even though thyroid is supplied to them and their physical development is aided, their mental development is arrested and they remain subnormal in their intelligence ability all their lives.

My friend the judge needed no further convincing and we went on from there to successfully conclude a weight-reduction program.

But I've run into another problem in trying to show patients why they could not possibly be victims of an underactive thyroid. The dress designer I mentioned previously told me she had proof that she was suffering from a thyroid deficiency and therefore

33

there was every reason to believe that her obesity was caused by that condition.

"Why, I've had several basal metabolism tests and in each case the result was between minus-20 and minus-30."

Translated into layman's language, this meant that the Basal Metabolism Reaction test showed that she used up energy more slowly than normal. This was used as proof that food she ate "burned" more slowly and therefore turned to fat more rapidly.

Unfortunately, under most circumstances the basal metabolism test is worthless. More and more physicians are beginning to realize that these tests are quite inaccurate, especially when not done at a hospital, and even then under particular circumstances and checked at least once.

The BMR test was developed originally on the assumption that the patient being tested would be at "basal" conditions; that is, at the state where the body is only producing enough energy to keep the vital functions operating. The only ideal circumstance for taking the test is *immediately upon awakening in the morning.*

After a patient has dressed, taken a taxi to his doctor's office and had to lie down for an hour to rest, it is not the time for the test. Yet this is how it is most often performed. The amount of mental energy expended, principally worry, during the time from awakening to the time the test is started, can be immeasurably great.

It begins when an uncomfortable contraption is clamped down over the patient's mouth and he is told to breathe oxygen in and out for a while. He wonders about the mysterious adjustments that are going on all during this time and this upsets his system.

Nearly all doctors disregard a basal metabolism test if it does not coincide with their clinical findings and observations. The doctor may repeat the test and still disregard the results. In my own experience I have found that a basal metabolism test is all but worthless except under laboratory conditions.

The only near-reliable way to have the test performed is in a

34

hospital, immediately upon the patient's awakening. Then the test should be repeated on a different machine with another technician performing the test, for there are sure to be errors due to faulty equipment and to human failings in interpreting data.

Under such controlled laboratory conditions, the results achieved by a BMR test can be ideal. Unfortunately such conditions are impossible to achieve in a doctor's office or outpatient clinic. Therefore the BMR test is next to valueless in this instance and the results from it can hardly be taken to imply that an obese patient is suffering from this condition due to an underactive thyroid. The BMR test has proved itself of great value, however, in determining the effects of an overactive thyroid—which, of course, has nothing to do with obesity.

There are other glandular disorders in which "fat pads" are likely to be put on certain portions of the body. Aside from the thyroid, the pituitary gland—found in the brain—has often been blamed for overweight. One of the results of underfunctioning of this gland is known as Cushing's disease. This failing will influence the distribution of fat in a characteristic way on the trunk of the body as well as giving the face a moonlike appearance.

But even if a person is suffering from Cushing's disease—the most characteristic as far as endocrine influence upon fat is concerned—a diet will bring about weight reduction, proof that overeating and nothing else will produce the fat which is deposited in the body.

An overfunctioning pituitary gland may cause a gain in weight, but it will not be fat. Some of this gain is muscle; more calcium may be deposited in the bones and thus they become heavier; and the lungs and heart enlarge. An over-all weight gain is recorded, but not of fat.

Another malfunctioning of the pituitary will cause adiposogenital dystrophy, best known as Froelich's disease, in which excessive fat will appear around the girdle area and on the midthigh.

Treatment of obesity with thyroid and pituitary gland extract was fashionable some years ago. The results were generally poor unless combined with diet which provided a low carbohydrate intake, and then it was successful only with the few who were able to follow the diet rigidly. Many a patient told to take three thyroid tablets a day would double and triple the dosage on his own in the hope that results would be more certain and quicker. The end result was that the doctor would find his patient suffering from thyroid intoxication while there was no effect on weight.

Contrary to popular opinion, you can have an overactive thyroid and still be overweight. If there is a gland involved in obesity, it is the salivary gland! Your overeating has made you overweight.

Is It Metabolic?

There's no stomach a hand's breadth bigger than another.

Cervantes: DON QUIXOTE

THE SUFFERER OF OBESITY has become involved in a vicious circle—a sort of perpetual motion.

What happens is this: as you gain weight, you need more food to supply the energy your body "burns" to carry the extra weight. To stay at your present stage of obesity, you must eat more than you would normally. Actually, the food you now eat compared to that you would eat at normal weight is in proportion to your present weight compared with your normal weight.

I have had patients claim that they are overweight because they "burn their food slowly," or perhaps that "everything I eat changes easily to fat." Just as patients do who have decided their ailment is glandular, these obese persons are offering their doctor the free diagnosis that they are suffering from a metabolic disturbance.

Obesity is not a metabolic disease in the sense that there is some upset or error in the metabolic make-up of the body. The popular suppositions that food in some persons turns more easily to fat, that some do not burn up their food quickly enough, that others get fat on little food, or that some stay thin on a great deal of food, are not confirmed by any tests performed in hospitals or by any research. These excuses are as much a face-saving device utilized by the obese as is the claim of thyroid deficiency. You must not be all too eager to absolve yourself of responsibility for your overweight.

Of course you do not consciously lie to yourself about your gluttony. I have found that patients who come to me with these stories are usually quite sincere about their observations and truly believe in the main that their food intake is either normal or only slightly above normal in quantity or quality.

Contrary to popular belief, practically all scientific tests and clinical studies bear out the opposite observation. In order for a fat person to continue to gain weight, he must eat larger amounts until the food intake proportionately balances the surface area of his body.

A young newspaper man once told me quite simply, "Thin people are thin because they burn their food more quickly than fat people."

That was his excuse for being overweight. Knowing him as a man whose inquisitiveness would get the better of him, I led him to conduct a little research on his own. He came back chagrined within a few days.

"Doc," he confided in me in his own manner, "everything I've been able to uncover points to the fact that my theory was all wet."

I allowed him to go on.

"Everything I've read shows that fat people burn their food more quickly than thin people because the body has to supply extra energy for all the excess weight as well as for their normal body requirements."

This patient made the discovery on his own. With this obstacle overcome, it was a relatively simple matter to lead him to the realization of what caused his own obesity. Then followed a diet regime and results; his weight dropped from 265 pounds to a normal 175 in eight months. And he has kept there since.

The observations which this young journalist made have been confirmed many times. But while I was able to convince him how wrong his theory was, I have found that an unusually large number of obese persons actually influence their physicians into stating opposite conclusions in spite of all the evidence compiled by authorities.

Don't let your metabolism be *your* excuse.

The Personality Problem _____

Thou shouldst eat to live, not live to eat.

Cicero: RHETORICA

You NEED NOT BE OBESE.

It has been obvious for some time that the cause of overweight must be found in the personality of the obese patient.

Once you realize this you have found the key to help yourself, and your doctor, in the battle against avoirdupois.

Unless the basic personality problem is solved, the weight problem cannot be bested.

So important has the problem of obesity become that the United States Public Health Service began a study of this health factor in 1950, a study that took almost three years to complete.

Drs. Benjamin Kotkov, Stanley S. Kanter and Joseph Rosenthal, working at the Boston Dispensary of the New England Medical Center, conducted this obesity-personality study. They recruited 135 overweight women and, to act as a control group so that a fairly accurate means of comparison could be maintained, they used 80 women whose weight was normal.

Many techniques were utilized, including such well-known psychological tests as the Rorschach Ink Blot test.

40

What did the Boston doctors find?

The women in the obese group were much more repressed, they engaged in daydreaming more often and, most important, they were not able to tap their energies to achieve as much success as the normal-weight women of the control group. One of the fat women was on the verge of losing her job because she lacked the courage to speak up and tell her side in an office dispute, even though she was in the right.

As a group, the fat women were much more tense and anxious than the women of average weight. When angry they were inclined to turn their anger inward. The result was depression. One of the obese group had a demanding husband who was a semi-invalid. She catered to his every whim, but all the while she developed more tenseness and became more angry.

The investigation showed that the obese women were noticeably more preoccupied with themselves and were not at all sensitive to the reactions of persons around them. Consequently, if someone to whom they felt close withdrew friendship or love, they were considerably more surprised, hurt and shaken than a woman in the normal weight group would have been.

Women in the fat group neither sought nor promoted new friendships readily. The fear of failure was too great. One woman who tried to make a friend of a new neighbor quickly withdrew when the neighbor's young child candidly commented on the woman's excessive weight.

The overweight group members did not enjoy social relations and worldly pleasures as much as the other group. Tense and miserable, they regarded social occasions as painful experiences. Since the obese do not feel at ease in their clothing, few of the fat women gave a "clothing" response in the Rorschach ink blot test.

Neither education, intelligence quotient ratings nor marital status had any bearing on the corpulence of the group's members. And whether the obese woman was only fifteen per cent overweight or fifty per cent overweight, she still showed this neurotic personality pattern.

Psychotherapy, then, proves to be the only hope in setting up a pattern of diet that will succeed.

The Secondary Gain —————————————————

Thou seest I have more flesh than another
man, and therefore more frailty.

Shakespeare: HENRY IV

THE GENERAL PRACTITIONER of fifty years ago practiced a type of medicine the wisdom of which has been widely ignored with the advent of miracle drugs.

During the past twenty years, these wonder drugs, along with better methods of clinical diagnosis involving laboratory tests and X-rays, have reduced the average patient to a "disease" rather than a human whose illness is coupled with fears and anxieties.

I have often heard a fellow physician refer to a patient as: "Mrs. Doe, a colitis case."

It constantly shocks me to hear such a reference.

It would be far more preferable to have this case referred to as: "Mrs. Doe, who is worried about approaching old age, her husband's business troubles and her daughter's desire to get a divorce. She is suffering from spastic colitis."

In this way any doctor will know just what this colitis case is all about. By understanding the emotional forces at work in the organic disturbance, the physician can give the patient a great deal of help in improving the condition. After the emotional im-

43

provements are achieved, the work in righting the organic wrongs is simpler and more rapidly accomplished.

The old-time family doctor, although he did not have penicillin, generally practiced what today is known as "psychosomatic medicine." He recognized that one patient's migraine was triggered by her husband's infidelity, that another patient's backache was an unconscious protest against the drudgery of his work and his family's lack of appreciation of his efforts to support them.

In getting to know his patients and their families well, the old-time family doctor began to recognize that many of their complaints were the result of some emotional difficulty. Although he did not understand the underlying dynamics and psychopathology, he clearly recognized that counsel alone often resulted in improvement for many such complaints as headaches, backaches, skin conditions and upset stomachs.

This technique has been rediscovered in recent years in the field of psychosomatic medicine. Today, of course, we understand the underlying mechanisms much better. The results are more complete now because the advent of better understanding has brought with it better treatment.

The principle of the *secondary gain* is the cornerstone of understanding the symptoms which plague these patients.

A secondary gain is a symptom which proves to be of some advantage to the patient, despite the fact that the primary disadvantage of the symptom may be painful or troublesome.

A public relations counsel who came to his doctor with the complaint that he had a "sensitive" stomach, said he was greatly troubled by attacks of nausea, diarrhea and vomiting. Doctors failed to find any organic reason for these attacks despite repeated examinations, laboratory tests and gastrointestinal X-rays.

This man tried one physician after another because each time he was told that examination showed no reason for these disturbances. Not hearing a diagnosis he unconsciously wants, he may eventually wind up going to some cultist.

This man's symptoms, despite their discomfort, are of secondary advantage to him. He becomes the center of attention with his family, his associates and his friends. Sympathy is directed toward him. All his failures can be excused on the ground that he is a sick man.

Yes, the man suffers physically. But he unconsciously revels in the role of an invalid. Responsibilities are taken away from him. But even if he must accept a few responsibilities, no one expects much of him.

Obesity is just such a secondary gain in the case of many overweight persons.

Although they may consciously dislike their unsightly fat, it does offer some advantages. For some it is a refuge—what we previously outlined as the *fortress of fat*. For others it serves as an excuse from arduous labors or responsibilities.

Most physicians have had as a patient a young woman who would be exceptionally attractive were it not for her unsightly excessive fat. This girl complains bitterly about her lack of social success or her inability to get fashionable clothes because of her girth. Most important, she is quite sad about her lack of success with the opposite sex.

One of the most unusual cases of secondary gain in my experience is that of an attractive young woman whose fear of pregnancy made her put on ugly amounts of excess fat so that she would not interest the opposite sex.

The daughter of a well-to-do Manhattan family, this girl was dominated by a mother who constantly harped on how dreadful childbirth had been.

"I am the only child," the girl told me, "and my mother's constant harangue about the pains of labor and the heartaches and headaches of bringing me up must have made a deep impression on me.

"Other than that, Mother had little to talk to me about. She had her own activities with Ladies' Aid groups at the church and her own circle of friends. She seemed to care little for what happened to me.

"I guess that's why I started eating more than usual when I was in my early teens and going to high school."

The young woman was quite correct in her analysis. In her hope to attract attention from her mother and to discourage attention from men, she put on weight. As she became fatter, she found she was less attractive to her schoolmates and she overcame this by becoming a "girl Friday" for a number of extra-curricular groups.

"I remember the kids used to call me 'Fatty.' Later, when I began to hang around bars I got such names as 'Fat Stuff' and 'Blimp.' I guess I became used to it because I don't seem to recall taking offense."

In spite of the fear of pregnancy instilled by her mother, the young woman still possessed deep within her the natural feminine desire to conceive a child. After graduation from high school, the unconscious fear and yet desire for pregnancy added to her craving for food. She soon was a not-very-neat 218 pounds with a desire for friendship which she went far afield to fill.

Loneliness led her to a Third Avenue bar—definitely not one of the better East Side category—a few blocks distant from her family's Sutton Place apartment. There she became a fixture and a friend to all.

"I had often overheard myself referred to as 'somewhat of a tramp,' and even that didn't shock me too much. After all, I had taken to not going home for the night quite often and awakening in cheap hotel rooms or furnished flats with one 'friend' or another.

"The day I realized I was pregnant, I could have died. I feared being discovered and, by means so devious I don't know how I managed, I learned the whereabouts of an abortionist. Fortunately, he wasn't a 'butcher.'"

It was a general checkup by her own physician some weeks

after the illegal operation that led this girl to wonder if she couldn't lose some weight. She had tried several diets she read about in magazines and newspapers and her doctor had prescribed "will power and diet."

"Will power" just wasn't enough, for there was no basic understanding by this girl as to why she was fat. When some months later her own doctor suggested she visit me, she came almost disbelieving that she could lose weight. Our first session gave me a great deal of insight with regard to her problem. She talked about herself, her home, her parents. The next time she told me of her friends, her bar escapades, more about her mother, and her abortion.

It wasn't hard to show her how the long tirades her mother had directed at her, regarding the pain of childbirth and the trouble of raising a child, had developed an unconscious fear of marriage and pregnancy. This fear expressed itself in her overeating and being unable to lose the excess weight—a defense against any man wanting to marry her. But, despite her fear of pregnancy, she became pregnant. The coexistence—either conscious or unconscious—of feelings or attitudes of love and hate toward the same person or object is known as ambivalence. Her ambivalent attitude toward pregnancy led her into obesity, illicit sexual escapades and, finally, unwanted pregnancy itself.

Paradoxically, she became a "party girl," an "easy" date, for the simple reason that it helped her to make new friends and to be loved for herself as she should have been loved by her mother.

Once she understood the reason for her fears and the cause of them, treatment became a simple matter. Within eight months she had dropped to 148 pounds and, with this physical transformation, came a spiritual one. Her reserve came to the fore and she was no longer the jolly easygoing girl of the Third Avenue escapades.

She blossomed into a mature and interesting woman, moved in circles more closely related to her background and met and married a man who probably would not have looked twice at her a year before.

Understanding is the prerequisite to a solution of the problems of obesity.

Obesity Is a Neurosis ————————————

*Obesity is a mental state, a disease
brought on by boredom and disappointment.*

Cyril Connolly: THE UNQUIET GRAVE

"WHAT DO YOU MEAN, I'M A NEUROTIC?" asked an advertising agency executive with an offended tone and look.

I knew immediately what was going through his mind. *This man*, he undoubtedly thought, *thinks I'm crazy!*

What an ugly word, and what an ugly thought. "Crazy," "insane," "mad," and many of the other words denoting the same state have no application to neurosis. These everyday terms, though little describing the situation, refer rather to psychosis—a far cry from psychoneurosis.

There is much confusion in people's minds as to what neurosis, or "a neurosis," is. Before we go much further, and since I have stated emphatically that obesity is a neurosis, let us define the term. There must be not the slightest idea in your mind that, in being labeled a "neurotic," you are being insulted.

As a neurotic, you are pretty much an "average" person. There is probably not a person alive who has not some neurotic trait.

The term neurosis is, first of all, interchangeable with psychoneurosis. They mean the same.

A neurosis is a relatively minor disturbance of the personality. It is an exaggeration of a normal protective mechanism. Some small unconscious fear, against which you set up a protective barrier, becomes enlarged in the unconscious mind and the barrier therefore needs to be exaggerated as well. One result of such a fear-barrier reaction with which you may well be familiar in other people is hysteria.

The symptoms of neurosis are the result of a reaction to a situation, internal or external, which a person finds himself unable to manage by any other method. We all suffer from such situations. Regardless of the proportionate size of the situation which triggers a neurosis, it is because we cannot contend with the situation that we become anxious. The anxiety state into which we go results in the development of abnormal symptoms and subjective experiences. So the personality disorder develops.

Thus, without understanding and without even being conscious of the underlying reasons, a person can develop a neurosis which will show itself in such ways as palpitations of the heart, fear of enclosed places, or perhaps an "illness" which among other things provides a device which will help the person save face in an intolerable situation.

Basically, the neuroses are reactions to emotional conflicts. They represent attempts to repress and transform impulses which a person has denied himself. Aside from being abnormal solutions to the problems, they are most ineffectual as solutions. The tension built up by the anxiety state continues to persist and in turn expresses itself in other symptoms just as disturbing to the person.

So disturbing, in fact, can these symptoms become that they can force a person to leave employment, to break off friendships and to avoid normal social contacts. Such symptoms may express themselves as upset stomachs, "lumps" in the throat, headaches and backaches. In fact, most patients seen by physicians, regardless of the purpose, tell of complaints which arise from a reaction to some intolerable situation in their lives. These symptoms are the unconscious protest against this conscious situation.

A neurosis, then, offers a person "symbolic escape" from a conflict.

The neurosis of a patient contains the clue to the nature of the underlying emotional illness. It serves as an unconscious safety device by which the patient can maintain some contact with reality. The reaction of anxiety, which is most prevalent, will alert a patient to danger. The emotionally healthy person will be able to turn his anxiety state into constructive use by recognizing it as a danger signal and following the warnings by effecting changes in the disturbing life situations. Emotionally immature persons all too easily become victims of their chronic state of anxiety.

The reason so many persons appear to link *neurosis* with what is generally thought of as insanity, is that they confuse the word with *psychosis*.

The psychotic person is one whose personality is almost completely disorganized; that of the neurotic is not.

The psychotic has no emotional contact with the real world; the neurotic is quite aware of reality.

The psychotic cannot differentiate between his subjective experiences, that is, the experiences he imagines and believes he is involved in—the "daydreams"—and reality.

The psychotic may have various sensory hallucinations and be unable to differentiate between imaginary voices and those of persons with whom he comes in contact.

The neurotic—that is, the "average" person, you and I to some degree, in some fashion—is fully aware of the external world and realizes all its values. On the other hand, the psychotic creates his own world and ignores reality.

While the psychotic doesn't even know he is ill, the neurotic person is greatly interested in getting well—even though within him all the forces of the unconscious act against this.

Neuroses have been classified into five major types:

Conversion hysteria which manifests itself with a physical symptom such as functional paralysis.

Obsessive-compulsive state in which precise and ritualistic acts are performed, such as children do in avoiding cracks while walking on a sidewalk.

Neurasthenia in which fatigue is the outstanding symptom.

Hypochondriasis in which the patient constantly suffers from various imaginary illnesses.

Anxiety state, the main category in which we are interested. This has been termed "the neurotic symptom *par excellence.*" It apparently is encountered as the basic symptom in all neurotic patients.

Generally, neurotic patients have a mixture of these types. Many psychiatrists feel that using one of these basic classifications is unnecessary and artificial as each patient is an entity unto himself to be judged solely on his own symptoms.

As for obesity, in most cases the prevalent feature is repressed anxiety.

There are, of course, as many mixed features in obesity as there are in any case of neurosis. Some obesity cases have many features of obsessive-compulsiveness, others have hysteria as a principal component, still others have symptoms of hypochondriasis, while disturbances of character and adjustment are in the foreground of others.

However, in most cases, it is an anxiety—which is unconscious and "buried under fat"—that is the main component of the obesity neurosis. The compulsion to overeat cannot be explained in any other terms. The obese person has a drive to eat far beyond that necessary to replenish the body's needs.

I have had innumerable patients tell me that they eat even when they are not hungry. Some have gone as far as to declare that they don't enjoy food.

Others find rich foods extremely pleasurable to the point of

52

eroticism. This latter group often has abnormally poor sex drives and complains of frigidity and impotency.

There are patients who eat incessantly and are almost unconscious of what they are eating, their attention being directed to other things at the time, such as reading or watching television.

Overeating provides a cloak for much latent anxiety, or it acts as a substitute for some deprivation in another area of life. There has been an attempt made recently to attribute this compulsion to overeat to a neurological or physical basis. Dr. Norman Jolliffe of the New York City Health Department coined the word "appestat" in an effort to explain the compulsion.

Dr. Jolliffe has stated that the appestat "is an automatic mechanism that when working properly, keeps the body weight and food intake in dynamic balance." He claims that the appestat is located in the hypothalamus, an area lying at the base of the brain near the pituitary gland.

Dr. Jolliffe has utilized the results of experiments with rats which have shown "that when this area of the brain is damaged, they (the rats) become food drunkards. They will eat everything in sight and soon become twice as heavy as normal rats."

Thus, Dr. Jolliffe claims, obesity can be controlled by "resetting" the appestat just as you would the thermostat of a furnace. This resetting, he claims, can be accomplished by six weeks of strict attention to a diet without cheating.

However, Dr. Robert H. Williams, in his contemporary *Textbook of Endocrinology*, has stated that while "investigations have demonstrated that lesions of the brain in the hypothalamic area are regularly followed by a development of obesity in rats ... perhaps of more importance is the failure to produce obesity in the other mammalian species in which the thalamus is injured."

Dr. Williams tells of an experiment with a large number of monkeys and says that "the negative results obtained ... cast a good deal of doubt on the proposition that hypothalamic lesions in humans are the actual cause of obesity that is sometimes seen

53

in patients afflicted with diseases of that portion of the brain."

Perhaps there is an appetite-control center in the human brain, as Dr. Jolliffe contends. Perhaps it is located in the hypothalamus. But, if the "appestat" does exist, it is most likely a neurological trigger controlled by the emotional life of the individual.

In my own experience, I have never observed a dramatic change in a patient's demands for food after merely six weeks of dieting—or even six months of dieting—unless there has been insight and understanding by the patient of the underlying unconscious motivation of overeating and the obesity that inevitably follows.

Obesity results only from overeating. In some cases the overeating is the response to an intolerable life situation. In others, it is a compensation for pleasures denied to a patient in other areas of his life.

There are reasons beyond the patient's simple statement, "I like to eat." The understanding of what "liking" means to him involves an understanding of the psychodynamics which underlie the case. That is to say, liking or disliking results from some facet of the personality.

The development and direction of a personality from childhood onward will determine whether a person will face life in a realistic and mature manner or whether one neurosis or another will develop as the answer to his problems.

Although every one of the obesity patients I have treated has shown the presence of anxiety features, I will tell you about one woman who was quite typically an almost pure "anxiety neurosis" case.

This woman came to me suffering from seventy pounds of excessive weight. Today, after several relapses, she is holding her weight at a level only fifteen pounds more than what it should be. The fact that she will not lose more weight is due to her resentment to the suggestion that she needs depth analysis. However, by superficial psychotherapy—that is, by allowing her to "ventilate" her troubles to me—she did acquire enough insight to cut fifty-five pounds of excessive fat from her body.

At forty-eight, the patient had been menopausal for three years. She complained of hot flushes, excessive perspiration, depression, headaches and insomnia. These symptoms were much like those of involutional melancholia which may accompany menopause. But, after realizing that during the period of her menopause she gained forty pounds and by determining that the woman was one who had had breakdowns in all the other crises of her life—including the birth of her children—it was obvious that the symptoms were the results of an anxiety neurosis.

Her story was a common one. Her marriage was successful and her two children had grown—the daughter married, the son in his last year at university.

"I feel quite useless now," she told me. "With my children not at home, there just doesn't seem anything for me to do."

This feeling of uselessness extended even further. Her husband—as devoted a husband as a woman could want—was successful in his business and obviously a well-integrated person.

"He would be so much better off without me," she added.

"All I ever do for him is cause him grief and worry with my complaining. I just can't seem to stop complaining about everything that bothers me."

Seeking to determine the motivation for her wanting to lose weight, the answer showed an attitude common among persons of her years—fear of approaching old age. Her reason for wanting to regain her "slimmer self"—although she had been slightly obese since childhood—was to help her recapture her youth which now she felt was rapidly slipping away.

"There is enough to keep me busy around the house. Now that the children aren't there, I only have a woman come in once a week to do heavy work. The rest of the work I do myself, because I enjoy a clean and tidy home and much prefer to do the cleaning myself.

"One of my big worries, though, is not being able to spend enough time with my daughter. She just doesn't know how to bring up her children properly. These modern attitudes on child-raising grate on my nerves.

"It seems to me a classic example of sparing the rod and spoiling the child. Do you know that my grandchildren are not yet toilet-trained, yet one is more than two years old and the other is one.

"And the way she allows them to get sloppy dirty and doesn't even punish them is most annoying to me."

Regarding eating, the patient said she had no idea why she had a voracious appetite.

"As a matter of fact, I don't even enjoy eating; but I seem to eat constantly in spite of that."

When the block against depth therapy became apparent, the only thing left was to attempt superficial psychotherapy by allowing the woman to air all her troubles and allay as many as possible of her fears which had basis in reality. Then followed a rigid diet, hunger-curbing medication and injections of female hormones.

This strict pattern peeled off fifty-five pounds of fat in six months. In the two and a half years following, the woman regained approximately ten pounds on each of three separate occasions. In each instance "short course therapy" was used to bring her back to the weight she had achieved.

Thus, by treating a neurosis, we were able to reduce obesity.

More about Neuroses ─────────────────

If you wish to converse with me, define your terms.

Voltaire

"JUST WHAT IS A NEUROSIS?" is a frequent question asked by patients after they have been told that obesity is thus classified.

Simply, a neurosis is a disorder of the personality caused by immature adjustment to life.

One of the greatest obstacles to the achievement of maturity is chronic emotional disturbance. Persons who suffer from "painful emotions" constantly seek ways of dealing with this pain. Among the various solutions are what are known as the neurotic reactions.

An individual's personality is determined by all his life's experiences, especially those of early childhood during which time his complete behavior pattern is established. Emotional stresses experienced early in childhood may be stifled and forgotten, but the child's emotional responses are distorted by these repressed impulses.

The child senses that these impulses—be they resentment, hostility, aggression or guilt—are unacceptable and therefore represses them. But the impulses remain alive below the level of consciousness. They interfere with the subsequent emotional adjustment throughout life. Whenever they threaten to reach the conscious level, the individual expresses anxiety and spontaneously attempts to reach a solution which would put that anxiety to rest.

The devices which the individual uses to solve his problems determine the degree of his emotional and mental health.

The "primitive" desires of an individual are most often not compatible with the social attitudes and values of the society in which he lives. This creates a basic conflict which must be resolved. If it is resolved in a mature, realistic fashion, the adjustment of the individual's instinctive desires to the demands of society is adequate and makes for an emotionally healthy person. If the resolution is immature, or is not completed, the result is tension and the creation of a neurosis.

One of the most common unconscious mechanisms which an individual will utilize to deal with an emotional conflict is *repression.*

Desires and impulses which are incompatible, or painful, to the individual, because these desires may not be socially approved, are removed from the individual's conscious awareness by repression. This process is never deliberate on the part of the individual. It is an unconscious rejection of an attitude.

All feelings of guilt or lowering of self-respect are most often repressed. For instance, the numerous sexual taboos which our society possesses may cause many women to repress their normal biological cravings. These women become prudish and hypercritical of many sexual matters in life.

Individuals with many repressions are likely to have many prejudices, especially against those who tend to arouse their repressed desires.

When a group of associated desires and ideas have been repressed by an individual, they become what psychiatrists term a *complex.* When repressions reach a complex state, any trivial

58

incident—perhaps only a statement by some person—which touches anywhere on this area of repression will arouse a violent response completely out of proportion to the "trigger" which evoked it.

The individual who reacts thusly will utilize a "good excuse" to explain his behavior. He will excuse himself because the real reason for his action is never consciously apparent to him. Thus, he begins to *rationalize.*

Repression often manifests itself as *resistance.* This is a common phenomenon observed in neurosis. It consists of the patient being unwilling to face the emergence of repressed facts. The patient then either retreats into silence or rationalizes his reluctance to face himself.

Sometimes the energy behind repressions is directed toward socially useful goals. This is known as *sublimation.* It is a part of all neurotic personalities who live happy and socially useful lives. For example, we all know of the elderly spinster, repressed because she was never able to marry and have children, who has found completeness, social usefulness and happiness in teaching young children or in welfare work.

There are instances where an individual who possesses a real, or sometimes only a fancied, inadequacy—either physical, mental or social—tries to measure up to the "standards" of society. They generally overdo things and their behavior becomes exaggerated. They are said to suffer from *overcompensation.*

The most common prototype of this symptom is the so-called "Napoleon" type—small men with overwhelming egos. They often use overloud tones when speaking and dress in exaggerated fashion.

The drive for wealth, prestige and power in many individuals is the result in most cases of a feeling of inferiority. It is overcompensation.

There are many conspicuous traits, either inappropriate or exaggerated, which are reactions to forbidden drives. Oversubmissiveness, politeness and oversolicitude may be expressions of unconscious anxiety, guilt and insecurity, just as overaggressiveness and belligerence may be an overcompensation for unconscious insecurity.

When repressed, undesired facts push into the consciousness of an individual because of the dynamic character of these facts, but take on a disguised form—a symbolic form—the process is termed *symbolization*.

The patient always is unaware of the meaning of the symbols which may take the form of dreams, facial mannerisms, body postures or psychosomatic physical symptoms.

Projection occurs when individuals see in others the very faults they themselves possess—and disclaim—and become ultracritical of these other persons. The projecting personality has repressed his "offending" desires and is quite unconscious of them. The projection, however, is always a clue to the underlying emotional illness.

Another psychological mechanism is *identification*. It occurs for example when an individual attributes to himself highly regarded qualities in other persons. The most common example of identification are the "hangers-on," those persons who will associate themselves in some minor capacity with for instance an athletic team, a motion picture personality, or a political party. The triumphs of the "host" become the triumphs of the "parasite," the failures will cause gloom and depression.

In *conversion* is seen a mechanism by which some emotional problem is transformed into physical symptoms which may be painful or disabling. Its purpose is not consciously recognized by the patient. In conversion is often found a "secondary gain." The products of this mechanism include psychological paralysis, migraine headaches and obesity.

Understanding what the causes of these mechanisms are makes understanding of neurosis more intelligible.

Oral Satisfaction

'Tis not the meat, but 'tis the appetite
Makes eating a delight.

Sir John Suckling: OF THEE, KIND BOY

MANY PERSONS ARE OBESE because their emotional development was arrested in childhood at the stage known as the "oral-
erotic."

The blame for their obesity may lie with whoever was responsible for their upbringing. But placing the blame on someone
else does not solve the problem; it does not burn away the excess
fat. By knowing where the blame lies, however, the obesity
patient should find it easier to regiment himself to a strict diet and
overcome the arrested emotional development of his younger
days.

The psychoanalytic school of psychology states that the individual passes through successive stages of emotional development
until he attains "true" maturity. He may, however, have his
development arrested at any stage due to a hostile or unhealthy
environment.

Overemphasis on any aspect of child rearing by the parents—or
the nursemaids or the teachers—may result in a neurotic adult

who has never outgrown the demands of an earlier stage of his development.

In the case of obesity, the patient's demands for oral satisfaction have become excessive. The result is apparent and obvious. These patients stubbornly resist treatment because any weight reduction regime is merely temporary.

They will try any faddist diet, for these at least will offer some indulgences in their oral drives. Rarely do these diets subject them to much deprivation.

At times, other motivations may temporarily assert themselves so that these persons will attain a normal weight for a short period. Unfortunately they can only reduce successfully and stay normal with mature understanding—that is, emotional understanding—of their oral drives. Otherwise their successes are short-lived and their weight bounds up to unreasonable limits again and again. The "caged demon" of oral eroticism reasserts itself in overeating. Sometimes, the patients will put on more weight after each diet regime and thus only continue to become more and more ungainly as they indulge their oral eroticism.

Let us go back to the very birth of the child so that we can understand what oral eroticism is all about.

When born, the child is conscious only of itself. It is auto-erotic and narcissistic—all its interests are directed to itself and its body. The interests limit themselves to food, defecation, sleep and alleviation of any painful body sensation.

In sucking a breast or the nipple of a bottle, the baby quickly becomes conscious of pleasurable sensations around its mouth. These sensations develop through three stages—*suckling, biteling* and *chewling*—as the infant learns to use the mouth to better advantage.

Many children, however, are reluctant to give up the very basic pleasure of the suckling stage and it will persist in thumb-sucking or other similar traits. Child psychologists claim that undue attention should not be called to this habit for it will disappear in the process of maturity. If too much fuss is made about it by parents or nurse, the child may persist because it is an attention-getting device. It creates an atmosphere of discord in which the child is the center and the child will then place a high value on this apparently undesirable habit.

If the home atmosphere is kind, permissive and tolerant so that the child has an opportunity to rid itself of hostility instead of repressing it, the child will give up his oral or other drives at the proper time.

At a later date, the desire for sweets—candy, chocolate, ice cream—will come to the fore in satisfying the individual's oral-erotic drives. You must realize, however, that these sweets—or whatever the individual will take to at a later date—taste "good" because they stimulate the oral-eroticism. They do not taste "good" simply because of their pleasant taste.

Most obese persons retain this desire for sweets or other rich foods well into the years of their maturity and sometimes for the balance of their lives.

The middle-aged woman who can sit down during an evening and consume an entire box of chocolates may claim that she "just adores" sweet things and can't do without them. Society condemns this sort of gluttony, perhaps because of the unconscious recognition that it represents something erotic and sexual.

An obese individual may rationalize the desire for sweets by stating that "I can't help it because I have a sweet tooth." That the person can't help it is true—the unconscious controls the mechanism. In essence this is a descriptive way of alluding to the process. But like all rationalizations it is merely an evasion.

At times the desire for sweets is an unconscious wish by the adult to return to that period of infancy when all wants were catered to by doting parents. This retreat from reality is present in all neurotics in some form or other.

The acceptance of reality and the making of terms with it is the sign of the mature individual.

63

Oral drives are not only manifested in desires for food. The need to smoke—cigarettes, cigars and pipes—is exactly the same. These items become a substitute for the comfort of the maternal breast or the feeding bottle which the unconscious remembers from infancy.

A good many smokers will laugh and think this explanation far-fetched. It is not. The reasons a person "likes" to smoke and "likes" to eat go much deeper than just the "like." The reasons for "liking" are based on associations which may tend to alleviate anxiety or cater to a system built on the basis of a neurotic complex.

The "likings" people have for sweets, for smoking, even for kissing, are normal in the sense that they are socially approved of in moderation or in that they become the accepted custom in the society in which the individual lives. But excesses or perverse forms of any oral drive are based on neuroticism.

The orality of the child still is seen in thumb-sucking. But the child often is willing to forego the oral satisfaction and physical need of eating in order to achieve the more dramatic satisfaction of being in the center of his parents' discussion, threats and bribes.

One result of oral eroticism in perversion is, in some cases, the denial of food by a child or adult. A way in which this can arise is through the overeagerness of parents to persuade a child to eat because the child may be "wasting away" or because food is expensive and troublesome to prepare. What happens is that a perverse refusal is created in the child with regard to eating. In this way the child recognizes its power to dominate its environment.

In adults you will often find the asthenic type who eats little, eats without relish and has aversions to many kinds of food. These persons often have repressed their oral drives out of a sense of disgust with the sadism inherent in the desire to eat.

To some, orality is unconsciously associated with sexuality.

Thus it is disgusting and unacceptable, and therefore it is repressed.

The universal motivation of all oral eroticism is seen by the prevalence of obesity. So widespread is the result of overeating that at least one-fifth of the huge population of the United States is estimated to be overweight.

One person who came to see me for treatment because he was ashamed of his excessive weight and ungainly physique is a man whose oral-erotic drive to eat is so great that, though he has been able to reduce to a normal weight several times in three years, he is a constant backslider.

I shall call him Peter. Perhaps you know him. He has been accompanist to countless singers in concerts, for he is an accomplished pianist and he has established a reputation in the music world as an accompanist who can help "make" a rising artist.

Peter's own words—"I like good food; well-prepared food. I like nothing better than a good meal"—sum up the entire emotional picture of his problem. To him food is like alcohol to a drinker, for whom one drink is too many and one hundred drinks are not enough.

Peter, an only child, was born in the "deep South" shortly after his father went with the American Expeditionary Force to France in 1917. His father was killed in action and his mother died soon after giving birth. Peter was brought up by his maternal grandparents whom he worshiped. He still lives with his grandmother whenever he takes a vacation from concert work.

"My grandparents loved me, I know, but they were very strict," he told me. "They had old-fashioned ideas about child rearing, and were careful not to spoil me.

"I remember being a willful child and throwing a good many tantrums. And I know that I was a bed-wetter until I was at least six years old, despite the fact my grandmother tells me that she was very strict about my early toilet training.

65

"But they soon knocked the willfulness out of me, taught me the traditions of the South and made a proper little gentleman of me."

The "proper little gentleman" grew into a tall, well-built person, who, while "chubby" as a child expanded to 265 pounds as an adult. He dresses extremely well despite his ungainly appearance, for his overwhelming interest in wearing apparel and style led him to select carefully tailored clothes, and he has spent much on maintaining a good wardrobe.

Peter is a bachelor. He has a wide circle of friends among both sexes and is regarded by them as jolly, witty and entertaining. His passion is food and he is an excellent cook in his own right—his specialty being Louisiana dishes.

While outwardly a calm person, he really is a bundle of nerves at most times. Especially is he so before a concert. He suffers periodically from insomnia and complains of violent pains in the stomach after huge meals. Doctors have kept him on barbiturates and antacids for years.

"I remember first being nervous when my grandparents sent me to a military school. My grandmother had taught me the social graces and I was quite well-mannered as a little boy. That and my chubbiness let me in for an awful lot of riding at the military school. It wasn't long before I was completely miserable.

"Added to all that I was utterly impossible as a soldier; I was just too awkward. And my athletic ability—if you could call it that—was practically nil because of my excessive weight. I couldn't even putt the shot or throw the hammer.

"I guess lots of things made me bitter at school. The taunts of my classmates were bad, but after the wonderful table my grandmother used to set, I think that the slop they served there was worse than anything. I still don't see how anyone could possibly do to food what they did to it there."

An interest in music, especially the piano, was recognized by his grandparents and he was permitted to take lessons off the school grounds. This was the saving grace. When he was graduated from the military academy, he passed entrance exams to a well-known conservatory in New York State.

With an adequate income from his parents' estate and the prospect of a "small fortune" at his grandmother's demise, Peter has little interest in making any more of a name for himself as a musician. He is a dilettante and has no real drive for success, though he has actually achieved a great deal of success as an accompanist.

Now in his mid-thirties, Peter has never had a true love affair or even shown any great interest in women. Although obviously not a homosexual, his lack of interest in heterosexuality has probably been on a superficial level due to a fear that he would be rejected by any woman in whom he might interest himself.

All through the three years Peter was my patient he had been extremely self-conscious of his excessive weight and his physique. He had made many unsuccessful attempts at dieting before he was recommended to me.

As a patient I found him most intelligent and appreciative of the emotional causes of overeating. His insight was, however, at a superficial intellectual level and he displayed a strong block against psychoanalysis. In fact he utilized several rationalizations so that he could avoid subjecting himself to therapy. He could never project himself into feeling any strongly charged emotional situation, for he preferred to stand aloof with a superior air.

He seriously tried to get into a regime where he would lose weight and hold himself at the lesser weight level. But, while accomplishing the first half of the program, he always failed at the second. Once started, his appetite was insatiable, but he was able to keep to the diet regime prescribed as long as he was given encouragement.

On four occasions during this period of three years he lost weight—once as much as sixty younds. Despite his backsliding, his enthusiasm never flags. He still is convinced that the "next time" he will succeed, and so, he rationalizes, he does not need depth analysis to help him.

This man, like so many others, owes his problem to his upbringing in childhood. No regime can help anyone who will not try to understand his own problem.

S'mother Love ————————————————

A child may have too much of mother's blessing.

English proverb

DIRECTLY OR INDIRECTLY, your mother played a major role in your obesity!

We must put the blame on parents—"Mom" essentially, although fathers are not blameless—but it is with pity rather than with anger. For if your mother, your father, or both, had not had so many emotional problems, you would not have grown up to echo them.

There is no doubt that the start of the problem of overweight lies in childhood. While obesity itself often starts in childhood, the problem can develop in later years from the same root.

No matter when you started to become obese, the emotional root of your "disease" lies somewhere in your childhood.

An understanding of the overweight child will probably give many persons insight to the over-all problem.

In families with obese children great emphasis has been placed on food more often than not. Desserts and candy are used as rewards for good behavior. Conversation centers on table delicacies. The child easily acquires the feeling that food is the end and purpose of life.

" 'Eating to live' gave way to 'living to eat,' " one philosophic patient put it.

Studies have shown that the mothers of fat children are emotionally starved women. They generally are disappointed in their husbands. They worry about domestic strife. They often are disappointed in the sex of their children.

As though in compensation, they pour out a love to their children they do not honestly feel. In this effort, they "give" the most obvious things: food and protection—protection from the unpleasantness of work and from contact with other children who might "play rough." But with all they do give, these mothers fail to grant their children the most important thing they need: true affection.

The emotional starvation of the child who perceives the real emptiness of his mother's show of affection may lead to a compensatory increase in food consumption as though the child were trying to satisfy his emotional hunger by eating.

Dr. Hilde Bruch, child psychiatrist and pediatrician, has made an extensive study of childhood and adolescent obesity. Her research has disclosed many startling facts: Families in which there was an obese child were generally small, less than two children on the average; the obese child was separated by many years from his next nearest sibling; 70 per cent of the total of obese children studied were "only" children or the youngest in the family.

Dr. Bruch noted that older children often were unable to dress or undress themselves. These, she found, accepted a great deal of help from their parents as though it were a matter-of-fact thing to do. They had become accustomed to being waited on.

Obese children who frequently had been described by parents as "normal" often were found to be quiet and withdrawn—far from normal for children.

One instance was cited where a mother disapproved of the neighborhood in which she lived, although it was a respectable, clean area of the city. This mother refused to allow her son to expose himself to the other children in the neighborhood. She felt he would suffer not only physical injury at their hands, but would suffer "morally" as well.

The child, the mother related quite seriously, came home one day and used what she described as "bad language" in talking to his younger sister. This "bad language," she explained, was just the sort of thing she was afraid of in allowing her son to even use the street. The "bad language" was used, she disclosed only after a great deal of urging, when her daughter interfered with the boy's play. The boy had told the girl to "scram"—using just that word!

Of 100 children whom Dr. Bruch studied thoroughly, only 23 had acquired any degree of independent self-care in keeping with their respective ages. The others exhibited a marked delay in their ability as well as their willingness to take care of themselves.

Studies of the 77 per cent who fell into the latter class showed that innate physical disability was *not* responsible for any retardation in independent behavior. It appeared to be due, rather, to marked defects in their training and to a delay in their having to assume normal responsibility.

The guilty finger points again at "Mom," for this 77 per cent in the studied group were below the "norms" because of a basic distrust held by their mothers in the capabilities of their children. A frequent explanation made by a mother of such a child, when asked why she did everything for the child, was: "I think I do it neater and quicker!" Undoubtedly, but look at what has been wrought!

A desire to do things for themselves exists in all children. After they reach the age of five or six, however, they can gradually lose interest in becoming independent. If demands are made upon them later, they generally are so slow and awkward in attempting to carry out these demands that they become easily discouraged—

especially if "Mom" has still not realized the error of her past ways and becomes irritated by the offspring's slowness, nags at the defect and then continues to give a helping hand.

The lack of independence sometimes extended to every detail of daily life, Dr. Bruch's 1938 study showed. She disclosed that another expression of the immature level of responsibility was the frequency with which bed-wetting occurred among these children. There also was a lack of interest, or willingness, to take part in everyday duties around the house, an interest which other children start showing between their second and third years.

The idea of expecting some assistance from their children did not occur to many of the mothers involved in Dr. Bruch's study until the children reached the age of puberty. Then the parents were disappointed by the inability and the refusal to help which their children displayed.

As a rule, the children who were helplessly dependent and who had no household obligations made little or no social contacts and avoided active games and exercise. Their parents frequently were found to be unwilling to give up "protective custody" of the children after they had entered school. They continued to accompany them to and from school, even at an advanced age, while normal children long since were trusted with handling the problems of traffic encountered en route.

If the parents finally consented to allow their children to make the trip to school unaccompanied by adults, they would spend tense and anxious minutes at the window watching every step while the child remained in sight, carefully checking off every second of time which they knew would normally be consumed in making the trip.

One mother of an eight-year-old was bitter about a new teacher who would not permit her to come upstairs with the child so that she could help with the child's clothes at the classroom door. This same mistrust in the child's ability to care for itself was further expressed in the frequency with which these mothers dashed to the school to complain of alleged injustices done to their children either by the teacher or schoolmates.

Dr. Bruch showed that although these obese children were an intelligent group, there was a lack of interests and talents among them. Radio, television and movies played a paramount role in their lives. This desire for passive entertainment was in many instances coupled with a demand for food. In view of the intellectual development of many of these obese children, it was astonishing to discover how many were satisfied with the comic-strip level of reading.

Investigation of the emotional significance of food intake and muscular activity among these obese children revealed that the emotional values of these two factors were opposed to each other. Food was found to have an exaggerated value and stand for love, security and satisfaction. Muscular activity was associated for many with danger, threat and insecurity.

The excessive desire for food may be looked on as a compensatory mechanism which is called into play at times when the bodily integrity and emotional security of the child are endangered, Dr. Bruch concluded.

In my practice, I have found that the mothers of obese children have often been ambivalent in their attitude. There has been a strange mixture of love and hate; the child, while grossly over-protected, has been the object of criticism and has been openly needled and shamed by expression of disgust and disappointment.

These obese children were not encouraged to be independent, yet they were criticized publicly and privately for their obvious lack in this respect.

A Westchester matron who brought her twelve-year-old daughter for therapy would not allow the child to say a word to me during the entire hour-long initial interview. For that matter, I could hardly make any statement of fact during that time without being interrupted by this aggressively talkative mother.

The child sat immobile and displayed no emotion whatsoever.

She stared at the floor. Within a few minutes her mother had relegated her daughter's problems to the background and was offering herself instead as a patient.

"After all," the woman told me, "I've had doctor after doctor tell me that Clarissa's plumpness is due to a glandular condition. And under those circumstances what can be done for her?

"Now I tend to put on weight for no good reason at all. Everything I eat seems to turn to fat, and if something isn't done about it soon, why I'm going to be almost as fat as Clarissa."

Poor Clarissa sat there much like a puppet. Her eyes betrayed nothing. They were cold and emotionless. Yet the mother's dismissal of her daughter's problem with the statement that "doctor after doctor" said the overweight was "due to a glandular condition" was probably untrue or greatly exaggerated out of context.

The next time Clarissa and her mother came to my office, I managed to get the child for a personal interview without "Mom" listening.

Clarissa was a greatly troubled and very unhappy little girl. She was approaching puberty—a time in the life of any young girl which presents enough problems without the added problem of "Mom."

"I often sit by the hour and wonder why I am alone," she confided in me. "I guess I just don't make friends—or don't want to make friends. But being alone frightens me and makes me very unhappy. . . .

"I guess I'm not very popular," she said later, and wisely added, "though I suppose I don't help matters. I guess a girl has to want to be popular if she is going to be."

We discussed a weight reduction program—and Clarissa was enthusiastic.

"Oh, yes, Doctor," she said, "I'll try very hard to follow any diet you give me.

"But I wonder," she added a few moments later, "if it'll do

any good? You see, I never really finish things after I start them. I like to do things, but somehow my interest dies out after a while and then I just stop when I get a yen for something else.

"I thought I'd like to play the piano a few years ago. Mother seemed pleased and I went to a music teacher. I guess it lasted seven months in all, though my interest in playing dwindled sooner than that. Mother's insistence that I continue made it last that long.

"Actually I found practice very tiring. I guess it was a little boring, too. I wanted to play more pieces right away, but there was so much tedious exercising."

We got onto the subject of her other parent and I discovered disappointment here, too.

"Oh, I adore Father. But he's never home often enough for me to enjoy him. His business keeps him in the city so long every day and he always seems to have to entertain other businessmen, so that when other fathers ordinarily come home, mine is still in the city.

"Gosh, sometimes I hardly get to see him on weekends. He has to play golf with people and junk like that."

On top of that, she finally confided:

"I guess my parents don't really love me as much as they do my brother Bill. Maybe it's because I'm so fat.

"Bill isn't so slim either, but he's in his second year at Harvard now—a real big shot. My folks are proud of him because he's such a good student. He's going to be a lawyer, you know.

"But," she repeated, "he's not so slim, either."

As far back as Clarissa could remember, brother Bill had been held up to her as a paragon of virtue in everything he did—especially in his grades at school.

"Mother is always scolding me for not doing as well as Bill did in school. I guess she'll not want me to go to college. And I think I'd like to go, although I might get tired of it after a while, too, mightn't I?"

75

Clarissa proved to be a good patient—for a few weeks. She came regularly and the weight reduction program on which I put her was proving effective. Suddenly one visit was canceled. It was the visit following an interview I had had with Clarissa's mother in which I tried to point out to the woman that the child's obesity was a reflection of the mother's attitude.

"No real success is possible until this situation is remedied," I said—putting it right on the line with a person whom I hoped might be intelligent enough to see that the results which had been achieved were the product of understanding of the surface aspects at least of the problem.

But insight was not accomplished with the mother—either because I failed in attempting to impart it to the woman or because the woman actually needed psychoanalysis before the child could be successfully treated.

At any rate treatment was terminated by the mother who obviously was resentful and outraged at the idea of my suggesting that she was anything less than perfect.

In obesity it is quite true that the sins of the parents are visited on the children.

Adult Immaturity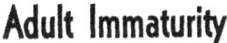

Men are what their mothers made them.

Emerson: CONDUCT OF LIFE

THE ADULT OBESE PATIENT is frequently an emotionally immature person.

Immaturity is found all too often today among adult individuals. Here again we must place the blame squarely on the shoulders of parents. As a youngster passes through adolescence into the adult years, the most important single conflict that has to be overcome is that between the desire to retain the protection of and the dependence upon parents, and the drive to achieve independence and freedom. The outcome of this struggle is influenced greatly by the attitude of the parents.

But while the blame may be placed on your parents, the power to achieve maturity may be obtained through the help of psychotherapy. There is no reason why you should doubt yourself, for you hold in your own power the ability to grow emotionally no matter how shaky a beginning you may have had.

The failure to attain a mature outlook is seen often in psychoneurotic personalities. Emotional immaturity is the cornerstone upon which a neurosis is built. But it is a cornerstone which a

77

"healthy building" does not need. It can be destroyed without causing the walls to tumble down. It is much like the cornerstone used in architecture as a memorial tablet. In this case the "memorial" is one of which no adult can be proud.

But immaturity is not a keystone. The keystone to the "healthy building" is maturity.

I have found that obese patients display many more neurotic traits than just obesity as the manifestation of their immaturity. They usually seek escapes into illness (headache, migraine, ulcer, high blood pressure and skin diseases), sleep, indolence, or procrastination.

They acquire these psychosomatic conditions or forms of running away rather than face the world and make terms with it. Instead of solving their financial, social or sexual problems in a realistic manner they become depressed or subject themselves to useless guilt feelings.

Many find an outlet in hypochondriasis. They will complain of palpitations of the heart, of headaches and backaches, of indigestion, or of countless other aches and pains. Thus, able to return to the sickbed, they can honorably resume their dependent status and enjoy the concern of their families and friends.

The link with obesity becomes obvious when many of the symptoms complained of by these neurotic persons vanish after they have had a good meal.

While hunger is a primitive urge to seek food and eating serves to relieve the tensions of hunger, by the same token, tensions due to nervousness, frustration, fear or worry can be temporarily relieved in the same manner—food. These tensions are described by psychiatrists as emotional reactions to unsatisfied needs—needs for affection, respect by others, success, social or economic security, and ease of mind.

In maladjusted persons, food will act as a relieving agent for these tensions. Excess appetite, then, is merely a reflection of this yearning. In a world which finds the obese person helpless in meeting the contingencies of life, overeating is an outward expression of an unconscious desire to solve all their problems through food.

They eat excessively because life is too difficult for them. Like the alcoholic's craving for liquor, their eating takes on a compulsive quality. And just as the alcoholic is unable to explain his compulsion to drink, so this type of obese person cannot understand why he overeats.

He knows that he is hungry—insufferably hungry. What he does not realize is that the strong compulsion to eat has nothing whatsoever to do with satisfying the nutritional demands of the body. Food is taken for non-nutritional reasons. It is taken as a source of comfort and relief from the tensions of emotional deprivation or for pleasure that would ordinarily be derived from other pursuits.

Eating makes the immature obese person temporarily forget his problems and unhappinesses. He feels "normal" in identically the same manner as the alcoholic finds "normality" and comfort in alcohol and the drug addict in morphine.

In normal people, hunger means a need for food. In fat people, hunger implies more than food alone. It is a hunger for security, a hunger for affection, a hunger for power, a hunger for happiness.

The sexual function is closely tied in with many cases of emotional immaturity. These patients are persons incapable of giving or receiving love. They unconsciously distrust the opposite sex because of traits acquired during their early, developmental years.

The Freudian school of psychoanalysis has much to say on this subject. This school links obesity with *oral eroticism*. That is, they believe obesity is the result of satisfying oral sexual cravings and is a regression, or failure to progress, from an infantile stage of psychosexual development.

Many leading psychiatrists feel, however, that although this theory has some merit, it is an oversimplification of a more complicated problem. Human motivation cannot in most cases be reduced to a simple formula, they claim.

Other philosophies have developed in the last half century—but a discussion of their relative merits is unimportant here. Suffice it to say research has shown that many obese patients have deep-seated sexual problems. Male impotency and female frigidity have been the symptoms for which many overweight persons have gone to physicians for help.

In many cases it has resolved itself to the classical problem of which came first: the chicken or the egg? Is the sexual problem the physical result of obesity whereby a sluggish overburdened body cannot cope with even ordinary sexual activity? Or is obesity the result of a troubled life which has affected the sexual function?

Food and oral satisfaction in these cases become a substitute for unattained sexual pleasures.

A thirty-two-year-old broker and café society habitué who came to me because he was about fifty pounds overweight revealed after a few visits that he had had many sexual failures. These especially became more noticeable after the dissolution of his second marriage, at which time he also started to gain weight excessively.

"Of course, the blame obviously lies with my ex-wives and my girl friends," he explained by way of excuse for what he felt was a chink in the armor of his masculinity. "They have been most uncooperative."

John (let us call him that) is the son of a wealthy manufacturer. John's mother and father were divorced when he was eight years old.

"I had a series of tutors at home, but none lasted too long. We usually didn't get on well, and if I didn't complain to my father, the tutor did. In either case, the result was the same—he went and another took his place.

"Summer vacations were most often spent in Europe and

finally when some of my friends were going to go to schools in Berne, I decided I wanted to attend school in Switzerland, too."

Here, he said, there was a great deal of discipline coupled with understanding. He found himself doing some studying. He got along much better than he had under his tutors and he managed to do well enough to enter Princeton.

"Once I was back, I seemed to be on the same old merry-go-round. The first semester at Princeton seemed like fun, but my grades were poor and I got a warning at mid-term that my work had to improve.

"That, coupled with the prank I perpetrated at the start of the second semester, spelled the end of Princeton for me. I had tried to make a solo effort to steal the bell from Nassau Hall—in the best traditions of the freshman class—but when a group of other freshmen disguised themselves as painters and stole the bell from the administration offices' belfry right under everyone's noses, I felt I had to do something else to make up for the plan which I had no chance to put into effect.

"So, one Sunday, when the huge campus chapel was filled for an important guest who was to deliver the sermon, I rigged up a very human-like dummy, hanging by the neck from a length of rope.

"This I arranged to have slowly descend from a dark spot on the vaulted ceiling just as the speaker was about midway in his sermon. My calculations were perfect. The immaculately dressed dummy, head hanging as though with a broken neck, gently floated down as I released my end of the long rope a few inches at a time.

"It broke up the decorum of that session—and it resulted in the end of my Princeton career."

Both marriages fared no better than his university life—each ended early and both ex-wives are drawing alimony. His first wife mothered a daughter who was four years old when John came to see me. He seldom saw the child, but was proud of her, carried

81

pictures in his wallet and continually talked of things she did—some evidently pure figments of his imagination.

I found him a man who appeared proud of being well-dressed and of owning good things. The so-called "reputation" he allegedly had among women was one of the things he enjoyed most; it was the prime facet in an unobtrusive vanity he possessed. His name was an oft-mentioned one in the gossip columns of the press and his figure was a familiar one in café society circles where he was regarded as a "notorious wolf," and a "chippy chaser"—the latter his own description of himself.

But despite his "reputation" with the opposite sex, he displayed an overt suspicion of women.

"The way I figure it, they're all after my money. There isn't a one who can be trusted. Pigs is what I call them—even my mother."

Yes, he said, he "adored" his mother—but! There were undertones of resentment. He did not quite express it in words, though I sensed that he fully believed that his mother—being after all, "only a woman"—had cuckolded both his father and his stepfather. As for the latter two he expressed almost complete indifference and there was a feeling of contempt obvious in his tone as he talked of his "father" and his "dad."

A gourmet—and a gourmand—he none the less was distressed over the excessive weight piling up on his medium-build body.

"I always was a stocky youngster, but since my last divorce about six months ago I've put on at least thirty-five pounds. My friends are laughing at me, calling me the 'fat boy,' and I just don't like things like that.

"I don't mind being the butt of a joke, but not of a running gag of that sort. It's like a never-ending Olsen and Johnson show and I never cease being the straight man. Frankly it's become unbearable."

Also unbearable, he revealed, were his failures at sexual liaison. As I pointed out, he placed the blame on his ex-wives and current girl friends and termed them uncooperative. His taste in women ran to the statuesque, often women older than himself. Many were prominent in the performing arts, other were dilettantes. His rare successes were among the latter.

John displayed a dread of being ridiculed either by gossip or directly by a sexual partner. At the root of all his difficulties, he felt, was a physical lack or failure. It took some persuasion, but I finally convinced him to submit to psychoanalysis.

Some months after undergoing psychoanalysis, he returned to continue his obesity treatments. He admitted great enthusiasm about his improvement and was able to get down to normal weight which he has held since.

The combination of emotional insight and reduction of weight have made a far more mature man of John. He is less of a night club crawler and no longer a "chippy chaser." He has found his potency problem solved and no longer feels the need to prove his sexual abilities to himself.

The attainment of real maturity is usually the beginning of a solution to the problem of obesity.

Back to the "Golden Age" _____

The childhood shows the man,
As morning shows the day.

Milton: PARADISE REGAINED

HARKING BACK TO THE "good old days" seems a common failing among mankind.

But were they "good old days"?

When you get together with an old-time chum and start to reminisce, is it the cold truth you recall or memories greatly embellished? You have to admit that the harshness of actual happenings is usually blunted by time.

While for a number of us life has been comparatively cruel and hard in its many demands and responsibilities, our childhood was more or less carefree. In our memories, the lack of responsibilities of those days makes them days of unlimited happiness, longed for consciously and unconsciously. They are days of an idyllic "Golden Age" not unlike the "Golden Age" related in many folklores.

In the folklore of many peoples there is reference to such a time when our ancestors lived the "perfect life." A civilization on a tropical isle where the climate is perfect, where fruit waits to be plucked and where the streams abound with fish and the

84

forests with wild animals—this has been an almost universal dream of things which were and which might be. In this idyllic spot there are no cares, no worries and all work is done by handsome, golden-tanned natives. But, our folklores tell us, our ancestors apparently fell in disgrace from this peaceful way of life.

Just as the unconscious desire to reach back to the "beautiful past" is based on disremembered things, so the idea of the "Golden Age" is pure fallacy. Anthropologists have been able to find no evidence of such an age anywhere. For that matter it has been shown that the more primitive a society, the more rigid were the social codes with their complex system of taboos and totemic restrictions. The more advanced a society became, the simpler its customs and the less restraining its mores.

The "Golden Age" on the tropical isle is merely symbolic of our childhood. For childhood was a time when most of us lived in a kindly, protected environment. Even when some of us do not come from such an environment, time and conscious desires will mold memories so that childhood conforms to the general pattern of a happy time—the "good old days"—when kind and all-powerful parents took care of all problems.

Many neuroses are the result of an attempt to retreat into childhood, or the inability to emerge emotionally from childhood. Many of us long for the security of childhood. This longing will express itself in many ways.

In obesity, it is seen in the desires for foods eminently characteristic of childhood, such as candy, chocolate, ice cream, cake, pie and desserts. Parents often reward or punish children by giving or withholding sweets. Obtaining sweets becomes for many children a sign of approval and love. They get candy because they are "good" boys and girls. Children feel most secure at moments of parental approval.

The child's desire for sweets is based on pleasurable taste sensations which are normally present. As the child ages and matures, if there is no neurotic disturbance, there will also be emotional maturity and this orality will be outgrown. Mature individuals do not have excessive cravings for candy, ice cream and cake.

Many obese persons are surreptitious chocolate and candy eaters because of a sense of shame about their gluttony. Others seek every opportunity to sample sweet dainties while visiting at friends' homes or on excursions to the soda fountain.

These "ashamed gluttons" will often go on a cake and candy binge after any defeat or disappointment they suffer. Their triumphs, however, are celebrated in the selfsame manner.

Many obese patients state that they "eat out of worry" or over-eat because of a celebration of some sort or other. The true mechanism behind this longing for sweets and overeating is generally unknown to the obese individual. It is an example of a longing for the "Golden Age."

The mechanism in these persons is much the same as that in pregnant women and their sudden cravings for particular foods. The mother-to-be usually gets these longings for something exotic —or difficult to get—at an ungodly hour of the morning. Her longing is based on a feeling of insecurity during pregnancy and an unconscious desire to test her husband's love. To prove that he would go through anything to please her, the husband wearily dresses and sleepily travels from one all-night drug store or delicatessen to another to find what his wife's little heart desires. Usually, when he gets back home triumphant, the desire has long since disappeared. But the test of his devotion has proved successful.

The longing for sweets in the obese is truly a longing for child-hood and the desire for the protection experienced from indulgent parents. Sweets, of course, taste pleasant on their own account, but the patient driven by such a neurosis does not know the meaning of "sickeningly sweet" or even of the word "enough."

Aside from sweets, a food such as milk has become symbolic.

Some persons often revert to a desire for milk when they seek to crawl back into the untroubled comfort of their mother's arms. The psychodynamics of this are obvious, milk being the original food.

The reason, therefore, a person craves certain foods is the symbolic nature of these particular foods which enhance the feeling of security in neurotic individuals. Obesity is often the outcome of this craving.

The hunger for sweets may in some few cases be caused by hyperinsulinism. Such a hunger can occur in a diabetic given an accidental overdose of insulin. There are symptoms of shock with pallor, tremors, extreme thirst and collapse. This extreme hypoglycemia, or insufficiency of blood sugar, is remedied by eating or drinking something sweet.

Some authorities claim that a similar condition can exist if the *Islets of Langerhans* in the pancreas secrete an excess of natural insulin. This would cause a lowering of blood sugar accompanied by all the symptoms of hypoglycemia. But I have never, as yet, discovered in an obese person a case of hyperinsulinism which can be proved by blood-sugar studies or glucose-tolerance tests. On the other hand, cases are legion where obesity has been the forerunner of diabetes—the very opposite condition to hyperinsulinism.

The craving for sweets in many obese persons cannot be attributed therefore to hyperinsulinism.

The cause must be sought in the emotional life of the patient. The identification of sweets with childhood and its experiences is an important mechanism.

Just such a patient was referred to me by a well-known psychiatrist. She appeared at her first appointment with a letter from the psychiatrist which read:

This will introduce Miss . . . who has consulted me because of tension, mild depression, globus hystericus, choking sensation and anxiety. Miss . . . has always been very highstrung and nervous, very aggressive and irritable. She has always been overweight, which disturbs her greatly.

Neurological examination revealed only a marked increase of the deep reflexes throughout (certainly on a psychogenic basis) and a tendency to overact to stimuli.

My diagnosis is that this patient is suffering from a character neurosis with reactive depression.

This patient is a strongly orally fixated person, but unfortunately she is not accessible to deep-going psychotherapy because of her limited intelligence.

Inasmuch as one of the factors in this patient's condition is her disturbance about her obesity, I am referring her to you for control of her weight.

The woman who sat across from me was thirty-four years old, five feet, six inches tall and weighed 280 pounds. Rather than refer to the psychiatrist's records, I had her tell me her entire story.

She had started to seek treatment a year and a half earlier after suffering a nervous breakdown following her father's death. She had gone into stages of severe depression and had become quite untidy in her personal habits. Her sister, six years younger and also unmarried, could not bear the patient's rantings and complaints and called in a physician who referred the woman to a sanatorium for psychiatric care. After three weeks she was discharged from the sanatorium and began treatment with the psychiatrist.

He found that after her mother died, when the patient was seventeen years old, she had kept house for her father and younger sister. She was quite obese then and, because of this, rather unattractive.

While she was used to a life of luxury, she was of only low-normal intelligence and had barely managed to be graduated from high school. Her father was a successful and prosperous building contractor who left his two daughters well provided for at his death. But though she had the comfort of money, a home and servants, she was afraid of life without her father. She distrusted all men and feared them. None, she felt, was like her paternal parent whom she loved with extreme devotion.

Because of her obesity, she had spent most of her adult life a recluse. Her interests were limited to television, radio, movies (of grade B quality) and trashy novels. While she hated her school days, she remembered her mother and father fondly.

She had been indulged in everything—parties, toys, even a pony. She remembered herself as a "cute, plump, golden-haired, blue-eyed child who was always made a fuss over" by relatives and family friends.

Her father, she told me, was a "strong, smart, important, looked-up-to and well-liked man" and her admiration for him was unbounded. To her he was the most impressive person a man could be. On the other hand, her mother she dismissed as having been a sweet person; she said she had been disconsolate "for some time" after her mother died.

Both she and her sister were always slightly obese as children but her sister did not develop so grossly. The patient accepted her younger sister with no overt like or dislike.

The psychiatrist's therapy had brought her a long way since her breakdown. One of the most encouraging signs was the building up of her ego in the therapy. She became cleaner and more tidy in her personal habits. She expressed a great interest in losing weight—for her most distressing personal problem was her obesity and she told of extreme cravings for candy, ice cream and "gooey desserts."

She felt that by losing weight she could become more socially acceptable and this was desirable since she admitted to extreme loneliness at times and wanted to make friends. Despite the therapy, she still was an extremely dependent personality with an unconscious longing to attach herself to a strong individual whom she could serve.

The strong motivation she displayed to emerge from her fortress of fat and find a real world again enabled her to lose eighty-five pounds in ten months. She was not an ideal patient for there was too much backsliding. Often she would go on candy and dessert binges, with much self-accusation and considerable weight regaining.

Her weight at 195 pounds still is not ideal. Many more pounds could safely be lost but it was felt that she needed time to live at this weight in order to absorb loose skin. It was also felt that the task of living and weight-watching at her normal level was at the time beyond her emotional and intellectual capacity.

But the success she achieved up to this point has been encouraging to her. She now wears more stylish clothes and, with her improved appearance, she is able to become an active member of her church in its various social and charitable activities. Though far more content than ever before in her adult life, she is still vaguely disappointed and dissatisfied with her life and wishes that some man—"not a fortune hunter"—would become interested in her.

The only real "Golden Age" is in a future free of the emotional problems associated with obesity.

The Fear of Fat _____

*Fear of danger is ten thousand times
more terrifying than danger itself.*

Daniel Defoe: ROBINSON CRUSOE

MANY AUTHORITIES FEEL that the only way to get obese
persons on the path to successful weight-losing is to throw a scare
into them.

I disagree. Fear may be an obstacle in the attainment of a
proper weight control program.

That is not to say, however, that an understanding of the
dangers of obesity should be withheld from the patient. It is
my belief that the overweight patient should be aided in reaching a mature approach to these very dangers. With this understanding, the patient then will find such knowledge an added
inducement in a diet regime.

The thesis to which I do not conform is that held by a number of authorities in the field of nutrition who have stated that
the only motivation which will force overweight people to lose
weight is fear. They state that such persons must be frightened
into dieting. Without this fear, they claim, there is not a strong
enough incentive present to accomplish the task successfully.

It is the belief of these authorities that merely informing a patient of the dire consequences of remaining fat will solve the problem of getting the patient to lose his fat.

There is no doubt as to the dangers of obesity. Some of those have been discussed earlier, but here I shall endeavor to list them comprehensively so that you may understand them and approach them with maturity and not fear.

While fear can never be the solution to any problem, the dangers of obesity cannot be overlooked. So well are they known, in fact, that obesity has been labeled "America's Public Health Enemy No. 1." Not without reason, for let us examine these facts:

As has been pointed out before, insurance company statistics show specifically that the obese do not live as long as they should. The Metropolitan Life Insurance Company has done yeoman work in this field, revealing that the death rate of "slightly overweight" persons as compared to those of normal weight is 22 per cent higher. The increase in death rate for those "moderately overweight" is 44 per cent. Those "grossly overweight" have a death rate increase of 74 per cent more than normal.

On the other hand, the slightly underweight live the longest.

In any illness, the death rate is higher for the obese than for the normal individual.

Arteriosclerosis, high blood pressure, diabetes, liver disease, heart disease and kidney disease are more prevalent and more serious in overweight individuals.

The obese are poor surgical risks.

Arthritic and orthopedic deformities are worsened by obesity.

That is an imposing list of "dangers" with which to contend.

In fact, it has been estimated that if all the close to thirty million Americans who are obese were cured, the benefits to the general good health of the country and the longevity of the nation would be more significant than if both cancer and tuberculosis were conquered.

With these facts explained in a mature manner you will find yourself more willing to undergo the task of losing weight. With these facts merely tossed at you in an effort to frighten you into reducing, you will surely increase your anxiety state and only add to the block which has prevented almost everyone from losing weight on their own.

The authorities who advocate the fear formula in the belief that mere knowledge of the dangers will be sufficient to turn the patient toward the path to reducing, are advocating a theory not unlike that of others who claim that merely knowledge of diets, of proper menus and of calories will be sufficient to accomplish weight reduction. Were that so, obesity would not be such a great problem today.

Knowledge is not sufficient without understanding.

Fear of the dangers only tends to worsen the problem. The psychodynamics of the anxiety state at the root of obesity have already been described. Patients who are obese have been overeating for one of three reasons: as the result of an anxiety which the fat cloaks crudely; or in order to substitute an orally erotic satisfaction for the pleasure they feel they have been deprived of; or to utilize fat as a secondary gain.

Even when a person is seriously ill and knows it, fear of the illness will do nothing more than add to the conscious and unconscious fears already present. In itself, fear will rarely provide enough motivation for the orally erotic individual to refrain from the substitute drive to overeat.

In rare instances will fear enable an obese person to give up a secondary gain which may be operating. For example, one patient who utilized his heftiness to get out of doing strenuous work and thus took from his shoulders the burden of being his family's breadwinner, willingly forewent this secondary gain when he first heard of the dangers of obesity. He was willing to start on a reducing program at once, though I continued on my program of helping him attain a mature understanding of those dangers so that the anxiety created by the fear would not result in another neurosis.

The obese should, of course, fear the physical consequences of their excesses. But too many of them overreact to this new threat to their security because they lack the understanding to put the facts in their proper light.

Without insight of the underlying emotional factors, it is too much to expect these individuals to react in a mature manner. As an obesity patient you are expected to face the world realistically, not as a place which can be molded to your own desires.

Not many months ago an elderly man, who as a successful publicist has to read as many newspapers and magazines as time allows, came to me when he discovered his obesity reaching proportions out of all bounds.

"I thought I was an intelligent person, and though I never tried to diet before, my portliness didn't really bother me.

"Some time ago I noticed in the papers and magazines articles on the dangers of being overweight. Because of my own problem I took even greater notice of them than I might have ordinarily, although in my business I read almost everything most avidly —you never know when some fact or other is going to be of value somewhere.

"No sooner did it dawn on me that my weight was an increasing danger to my life than I decided to do something about taking off the excess pounds. I began to worry about how many calories I was consuming every day—counting, charting and conniving to cut down.

"This sounded good to me, but somewhere along the way something must have happened. The more I worried about my obesity, the heavier I became. Now it's reached proportions that really have me scared silly.

"Can you imagine a grown man scared silly?"

It doesn't require any stretch of the imagination to see what an anxiety state this man had worked himself into. The reaction to the fear he had developed was an unconscious drive to eat even more. In effect it was only a retreat from the problem—a retreat further into the illness. This was a man who had always solved his problems by eating instead of facing up to them. How could he be expected, then, to face this new threat except by overeating?

A typical case of "the frightened man" was the owner of a garage who came to me a short time after he had been turned down for life insurance because of gross obesity and high blood pressure.

This came as a rude shock. Not too many years before he had been in the Army and had been classified as 1A.

"What I can't figure out is how I deteriorated from 1A to a virtual 4F in six years," he told me during his first visit.

"When I got over the initial shock, I began to look into this business of being overweight. I need insurance because I now have a family on the way and the insurance company doctor told me that unless I lost weight, so that my blood pressure would go down also, I didn't have a chance of getting a policy.

"What I read about obesity scared the hell out of me. Do you know how dangerous it is to be overweight?" he asked.

I sympathetically nodded and started on the preliminary road to helping this ex-GI.

His story was not unusual, but to outline the growth of a neurosis which the anxiety of fear only heightened, let me recount it.

Joe (let us call him that) was born in 1919, the only son of a weak, submissive and indulgent mother and of a domineering and stubborn father who demanded his own way in all things.

As an only child—and son—Joe's father expected great things of him. The father was a successful dress manufacturer and lavished his heir with gifts, but not kindness. In fact, he was utterly severe with Joe.

"My father always explained to me later that he was severe because he didn't want me to become a spoiled child, like all 'only children' turn out.

"Actually the strictness he showed toward me made me not only fear him but hate him as well. I can't help but hate the man for his continuous sarcasm and the countless beatings I got. Those outweighed any of the gifts he gave me.

"The worst of it is that I know that this feeling of hate is unworthy. A son should love and respect his father, shouldn't he? I certainly will expect it of my children.

"And I'm not incapable of love. I do love my mother. I always did adore her. She was always so understanding and good to me. If only my father had been a little understanding."

That set the pattern in childhood.

By the time Joe was twelve years old, it was the depth of the depression. Joe's father went bankrupt and, from the comparative affluence enjoyed by the family, they went to near poverty. Like many a man in that era, the father became an embittered person. He harangued Joe all the more and hounded him with the idea of studying for one of the professions so that he could attain financial security along with respectability.

Joe, unfortunately, was not one who was able to apply himself to his studies. His grades were average, but no more than that. This resulted in many quarrels with his father and only added further to the atmosphere at home which irritated Joe to distraction.

"My parents were bitter because of our reduced circumstances. We no longer ate as well, of course; many meals consisted of only spaghetti or potatoes, and bread was the staple of our diet where meat had once been.

"Come to think of it, I started to get fat by the time I was fifteen. I guess that it must have been all the starchy foods we were forced to eat, though that never occurred to me before.

"In any case, the more I quarreled with my father about my grades at school, the more I got to hate the place.

"Actually I first discovered my love for tinkering with engines then. One of the boys had an old jalopy and we used to tear it down every weekend. I mentioned this to my father and asked if I couldn't go to a trade school where I could léarn to do something I enjoyed.

"He became more sarcastic than ever. Mumbled for months about a mechanic's life being a difficult and unrewarding one. Wanted me to be a lawyer, or a doctor.

"So I finally managed to graduate from high school—but really the idea of going to college was frightening. I knew I could never get the grades necessary to enter a professional school and stay there.

"It wound up with one bang-up quarrel with my father. I ran away to California where I managed to get a few jobs on fruit farms, but when I wrote home and my mother begged me to return and said my father wanted me back, too, I came."

Once back home, the question of further schooling was not mentioned and Joe went to work at a filling station. There he stayed, learning a great deal, until he was drafted in 1942.

In the Army his troubles started again. A member of a truck company, he didn't get along with his sergeant and the company commander. He claimed that they constantly harassed him and ...

"I finally blew my top, but before I could do any serious damage I was shipped to the station hospital and thus avoided a court-martial."

He recalled that both the sergeant and the captain involved had called him a "fat slob," and related that his father had sometimes used that same term to him.

"I'm sure it was the use of that phrase that caused me to go off my rocker. If it hadn't been for the chaplain and an understanding medic who intervened in my favor, I don't know what might have turned out."

These two arranged for hospitalization with a diagnosis of "psychoneurosis, type undetermined." Two months later he was released and transferred to duty with another outfit, and served in the continental United States until late in 1946 before he got an honorable discharge.

"A chap I met in the Army and I got a GI loan and we opened a small filling station and auto repair shop. We did well and now we have a fair garage business in a larger place.

"Even though everything was going our way, my father still was critical of the place and skeptical of my being a 'mechanic.' Mom was encouraging and still is."

His mother also encouraged him to get married, though, by his own admission...

"I never was a man with the ladies. In fact, I never learned to dance until after I got married.

"Julie and I got married last year and we're expecting a baby in a couple of months. That's why I wanted to get some insurance. I had let my GI insurance lapse.

"Then came the doctor from the insurance company. A couple of days later I was told that I'd not passed their physical."

At the time he took the insurance company's physical he was sixty-five pounds overweight. Feeling that his "days were numbered" once he realized the dangers of this condition, he made attempts to diet.

"The more I tried to diet, the more I wanted to eat. I couldn't resist going to the refrigerator every night before bed—sometimes also in the middle of the night when I awakened with a ravenous hunger—and making myself a 'Dagwood' sandwich. And I had eaten three square meals during the day, too.

"I guess you know what happened, don't you? I gained twelve more pounds in the next eight weeks."

The idea that his father was right—"that I lacked character, that I was worthless, that I had no will power"—began to haunt him. A successful businessman who was known for his comparative joviality became a moody and introspective individual.

It was apparent that Joe had developed a severe anxiety state. The first thing it was necessary to do was to point out that his struggle with obesity was not a futile one, that irreparable damage had not been done to his health, that much could be accomplished and that he would not only get an insurance policy, but live out his allotted years in good health.

All his troubles with his father were aired. He had obviously been searching for the kind, indulgent, protective "father" in place of the cruel tyrant he had known since childhood.

With the easing of his emotional problem, he was put on a rigid diet, given vitamin supplements and hunger-curbing medication.

Joe did extremely well. In five months he lost seventy-two pounds. He became a good weight-watcher. Once, when he regained eight pounds slowly some six months later, he worked it off along with an additional four pounds.

Since that time he has held his weight well. He is quite conscious of his weight and claims that the amount of restraint he needs now to keep it at a normal level is "not too painful" to achieve.

Conquering the fear of fat is an essential in weight reduction.

Social Obesity

Fat, fair and forty.

Scott: ST. RONAN'S WELL

Do YOU RECOGNIZE this picture?

The time—about an hour after a rather hearty meal.

The place—a living room.

A member of the group—a rather obese person holding a canape in one hand, a cocktail in the other.

The topic of discussion—the latest effort at *reducing*.

Is it you? If so, then you have succumbed to the most common type of obesity today—social obesity.

Aside from the emotional and other factors which I have previously discussed, there are three factors in obesity which are of some importance. One is the anthropological, another is economic and the third is social.

We must recognize that even today there are cultures or societies extant in which fatness—especially in women—is regarded as a prime attribute of beauty. And while this is especially true in Eastern Europe, the Middle East and the Orient, it holds none the less true in some of the ethnic groups which comprise our North American civilization.

Only the other day a most attractive young woman complained to me that her "hips and *derrière* are just too small—they aren't sexy enough." Less than a half-century ago our civilization quite generally accepted the buxom form which Lillian Russell made so popular. It was the epitome of feminine pulchritude and vanished at just about the same time the glamorous singer herself died.

As long as obesity had "prestige" value, it held great vogue. The advent of the "flapper" era after the First World War, and the death of Miss Russell in 1922, however, contributed to the decline of prestige which corpulence once held on this continent. But our concept of feminine beauty—as delineated by the press in various aspects of dress and undress—even today is thought of as decidedly inferior by the average man of Eastern Europe and the Middle East. To him, his buxom, overripe charmer has it all over the American Beauty.

The attitude of these peoples, too, toward the obese man is one of respect. His impressive girth to them is a sign of affluence and importance. With such an attitude inbred in a culture, the emotional factors of obesity are no longer important as one of its causes. To these peoples, obesity is an attribute, not a neurosis. The herd attitude will create enough drive so that becoming obese is necessary in order to be fashionable.

In such a society, the neurotics will tend more toward asthenia rather than the other way. Their neurosis will be either an unconscious protest against the so-called norm of obesity, or will be caused by the same emotional factors which operate in any society. But the neurosis will lead to extreme thinness.

It might be noted, that, naïvely, Eastern Europeans and Orientals have long regarded obesity as an attribute of good health. The fallacy of this, of course, was only recognized in our civilization recently.

In societies where the economic status of the bulk of the population is marginal, obesity has become evidence that the individual is wealthy, and thus influential. This is obvious to the members of these societies, for food is not easy to come by.

In America, however, the opposite often holds true. Here obesity may be a sign of poverty, for the high price of meat and other protein foods means that the underpriviliged must rely on more reasonable carbohydrate foods. And while potatoes, bread, spaghetti and macaroni may be very tasty, they are also very fattening.

"But my obesity must be glandular, Doctor," said the large mother of a family of nine. "Feeding eleven persons on the small wage my husband earns doesn't allow for overeating."

This she offered after telling me of the foods she feeds her brood. The carbohydrate content of her family's meals would almost supply enough energy to power a rocket to the moon.

But even today there are many Americans who hold attitudes close to those of Southern and Eastern Europe in that they regard "plumpness" as a desirable attribute. These people look with resentment on women who are "scrawny and skinny."

In many families the dinner table is the center of everyday life. Food is the favorite topic of discussion. Great pride is taken in culinary accomplishments of the womenfolk. The men eat accordingly—staggering breakfasts and "man-sized" dinners. Children raised in such households will become as obese as their parents. But rather than blame environment for their obesity they will place the blame on heredity.

The culture we have developed in America has many special facets involving food and eating. The entertainment of friends and business contacts with food and liquor has played a large part in our social mores. Despite the custom of eating three full meals a day, visits in the evening to friends and relatives invariably mean being served liquor and soft drinks followed by a midnight "snack." This snack is often quite an impressive pick-up meal in itself, sometimes consisting of cold cuts, various salads, rich cake and cookies, and coffee.

One is expected to eat heartily lest the hostess be insulted, for she has gone to great trouble and expense to prepare this repast. Everything the hostess has done is observed with great interest by the ladies visiting so that they can in turn attempt to outdo these efforts when they entertain. This type of social competition is all too common. The attempt to be hospitable can easily grow into a monster as the lavishness in entertaining grows to extensive proportions. It becomes a test of prestige, financial affluence and generosity.

A hostess cannot be niggardly at her entertainment table for she fears the barb-tongued gossip of her friends.

While every hostess is concerned about making a good showing at the dinner table, she is also concerned about her slowly thickening waistline and rapidly spreading hipline. The once size 12 or 14 into which she fitted has given way to an 18 or a 20.

The fashionable hostess is expected to remain attractively slim while lavishing her guests with rich foods and drink. The hostess, too, must insist that the food be eaten, else it will reflect on her efforts and their financial standing and thus lessen her prestige.

What a vicious circle!

And, of course, the favorite topic of conversation while this food is being consumed is the current attempt at slenderizing. The latest victim of a lose-weight fad will sit, literally stuffing her face, and tell of her new delicious diet which comprises wheat germ and blackstrap molasses, and then, *presto*—thin.

The giving of food and drink to guests is an ancient custom. Its traditions are deep-rooted. It is a gracious custom because it is a symbol of affection. To give food and drink is to give love. But while it may be a desirable custom, it is desirable only for those whose neurosis is not rooted in satisfaction of oral sensations. Otherwise this extra food and drink will only help contribute to the excessive obesity of the neurotic whose drive is toward food.

For the neurotic whose drive is in other directions, this extra

103

food will be of little or no importance. These people merely make up for the overindulgence of food by foregoing enough food at times when they are alone. In this way they maintain a balance which adjusts itself every few days.

Serious dieters are often treated with amusement at social gatherings. They are cajoled into eating rather than having their intention to stick to a diet treated with respect.

Persons who have adjusted to a diet are doing a worthwhile thing for their own health and self-respect. This attitude should be emulated, not chided. The motivation may be solely one of vanity, but even if this is known there is no reason to urge such persons to break their diet, even once. The result of the diet will be a beneficial one. Don't deride it. After all, who is to determine where self-respect ends and vanity begins?

In many cases, social obesity in a patient is only a matter of ten or fifteen pounds in excess of normal, or desirable, weight.

This was the case of a thirty-four-year-old matron who consulted me after she had struggled back and forth over several years to take off fifteen pounds, often succeeding only to have it reappear. She and her husband, publisher of a small magazine, lived on Long Island, where they maintained a beautiful home for their two young daughters.

"Ever since the birth of my first child, I've been on this seesaw of excess weight," she told me. "I realize that I gain the weight at the height of the 'social season' and then can successfully take it off, if I make the effort, during the 'off season.' "

The woman was intelligent—a college graduate and former social worker—and understood intellectually all the possible motivations at the basis of her obesity.

"I have contemplated psychoanalysis," she said, "but somehow I feel that unless I can break the merry-go-round in which we move, that, too, will do no good. Actually the problem—as are all my others, I think—is minor."

Here was a woman, happily married, the mother of two lovely

children, a charming and successful hostess, with the character to make a success of her life and yet lacking the intestinal fortitude to break the vicious circle of reciprocal entertaining which leads to her overweight.

"With seven or eight weeks of dieting during the lull in the social season, I can easily get down to a desirable weight.

"But then the rounds of entertainment resume and there I am again, stuffing myself into a girdle and larger dresses.

"I've often thought that perhaps I should try to entertain more often. I don't have to eat when I'm at home, but I can't insult a hostess by refusing everything set down before me. Perhaps if I start having people in every night of the week, I'll have a legitimate excuse for not going to other people's homes and that will solve my problem."

Her facetiousness could have meant that the solution of her problem lay deeper than just in a change of social attitudes. The excuse of social obesity may have been only rationalization on her part. It may have been a smoke screen for more deep-seated difficulties.

None the less, despite whatever other problems may have been at the root of the situation, her social life was an important contributing factor to this woman's obesity.

At the other end of the scale we have a form of social obesity which hinges on economic factors exactly the opposite to those involving the Long Island matron.

The wife of a post office employee, mother of four children, consulted with me when she realized that the extra sixty pounds she was carrying added years to the forty-two she had lived.

Her excess weight started with the first of her six pregnancies. After each child was born, as well as after each of two miscarriages, she added weight to what was once a slender figure.

"I was married just after I got out of high school. I was considered a fairly pretty girl—and I was slender.

"We had our first child about a year later and after he was

105

born I gained about seven or eight pounds—permanently. That wasn't too bad, except that it happened again after the second child was born and it kept up with each pregnancy.

"Feeding a large family afterward meant careful management. So potatoes, bread and macaroni were important staples in our diet. Soon I was like I am today—with sixty pounds of useless fat."

This was the only real bone of contention in the woman's life. She was an excellent housekeeper and a good mother. Her home was clean, her meals wholesome and kept within the family budget. Her children were dressed cleanly and studied hard at school. She hoped her two oldest sons would become professional men.

"If only I could lose some weight. I don't like looking like a slob. I'm still young enough to be attractive and there's no need for me not to be."

The problem of losing weight here was solely one of diet. It meant difficulties—preparing three sets of meals daily: for her children, for her husband who worked a late shift and therefore did not eat with the family, and for herself to conform with her diet.

She felt uncomfortable about her diet because her foods were more expensive than those she fed the family. The diet called for high-protein food only. It disturbed her, as well, to make different food for herself than for her husband and children. But her husband enjoyed starchy foods and as a result was quite as obese as she.

"Tom thinks this dieting is crazy," she remarked one day after several weeks of treatment which began to show results. "He thinks it's a lot of nonsense. I've showed him the articles you pointed out to me about how obesity is a dangerous condition and cuts down the life span, but he just sneers at the whole business."

Her husband's attitude didn't help matters, but the patient

was a determined woman. She kept at her diet, balanced her budget to enable herself to buy the more expensive foods, and finally succeeded in permanently dropping thirty-five of the excess pounds.

The life people lead is reflected in their weight. A change in weight requires a change in the way of living.

Relatives and Friends

I see no objection to stoutness—in moderation.

W. S. Gilbert: IOLANTHE

THE GREATEST POTENTIAL ENEMIES you have in your battle with the bulge are your relatives and friends. They constitute an unwitting fifth column as they bore from within while you struggle with avoirdupois.

Just as you have to realize that your parents were partially responsible in the beginning for your emotional problem which has led you to put on weight, so you must now realize that you cannot trust most of your relatives and friends while you joust with extra pounds. They will not often be sympathetic. They will ridicule, laugh and sneer.

You must be prepared to disregard their "well-wishing" and go your own way. You are intelligent enough to realize that your physician's advice is far more competent than any layman's intended help.

If you allow your relatives and friends to harass you with criticism, defeatist attitudes and faddist advice, you will have a greater obstacle to overcome than just the problem of accepting the emotional basis of your obesity.

A recent newspaper interview with a Washington, D. C., writer singled this attitude out quite distinctly. This man reduced from 350 pounds to 175 pounds. But, he claimed, the most trying aspect of cutting his weight to half was not the sacrifices in restricted food intake. It was, instead, the attitudes of his friends which he described as "never helpful."

We have been accustomed to linking corpulence with comedy. The traditional circus clown is fat. In recent years, too, Hollywood has come up with several comic stars who capitalized on their fat to evoke laughter.

There is something in the make-up of the human which results in attitudes of derision toward the obese. Along with laughing at clumsiness, body and speech deformities, and unfortunate mannerisms, we are inclined to snicker at obesity. The laughter gathers a sense of comfort in feeling superior to a "less fortunate" individual. Persons who unconsciously feel limited in their lives have need of enhancing their sense of security by laughing at those they believe less fortunate than themselves. Studies in the psychology of wit and humor reveal this element of a feeling of superiority on the part of the audience amused by a comic figure.

So it is with persons who will deride your attempts to diet and reduce. In you they have a "comic figure," a "less fortunate fellow," an object of derision. If you allow them to succeed in their snide attacks, you have lost a good half the battle. If you can intelligently pigeonhole their attitudes into file-and-forget categories, you have won a major struggle and the final victory is yours to be won as well.

Patients often complain that their friends will not regard their obesity seriously and ridicule their efforts at dieting. Waiters in restaurants often prove uncooperative as well, and act amused when a dieter places an order. I have had patients tell me that they have had to resort to explaining to both friends and restaurant waiters that they are suffering from a diseased gall bladder and thus cannot eat fried, fatty and rich foods. They claimed this was the only way in which they could get any sympathy and cooperation from such persons who thought that obesity is funny, but that gall bladder disease is serious.

The irony is that obesity has far more serious implications as a disease than gall bladder disease, which is, as a matter of fact, often a result of obesity or associated with it.

Mistaken attitudes on the part of friends may upset your entire diet regime. You undoubtedly will have friends who will feel that you are suffering greatly because of your restricted food intake program. These kind persons will urge you to sample delicacies. They believe this sort of thing is an act of hospitality and therefore in your interest.

Frankly, these people are thoughtless! They can easily break down your most earnest determination at dieting. You must discourage them as much as you must discourage yourself from falling into the traps they set.

Such "friends" are no better than the well-meaning people who will offer a reforming alcoholic "just one drink—after all, one drink won't hurt."

You are also likely to encounter a great deal of sadism on the part of friends during your diet regime. In many individuals there is a streak of latent sadism, all too easily brought to the fore. Thus in your effort to lose weight you may evoke a great deal of cruelty on the part of friends. You may be subjected to kidding, a most common form of sadistic expression. And this kidding will be a hard thing to take after a while.

None the less, you must be prepared for this and do battle bravely.

The physical requirements necessary to a successful weight reduction program are Spartan enough without having the dieter subjected to practical jokes and ridicule. Some of my patients complain bitterly that their friends charge them with being motivated purely by an overwhelming vanity in their desire to rid themselves of excess weight. This form of ridicule is infantile, for vanity as a motivation in any area of life may be extremely worthwhile.

The desire to appear more attractive is a common thing in all of us. A clean-cut, healthy body, clothed neatly, is not an attainment which should be reprehensible.

Patients have complained to me that relatives and close friends have become "prophets of doom or futility." Instead of encouragement, they will try to show the dieter the alleged uselessness and unattainability of pound-losing.

They make claims that obese persons can never become slim because it is their nature to be fat. Sometimes they will admit that a little weight can be taken off, but they quickly add that once the dieter no longer has the assistance of his physician and his "reducing pills," he will quickly regain his corpulence.

Some of these "good friends" won't hesitate to tell you how "terrible" you look once you have lost weight, for there is a looseness of skin and an unequal loss at various parts of the body. The usual comment is something like: "Well, you've succeeded in losing some weight, but you sure look like hell as a result." The inference is that your health has been impaired in some manner.

You must understand clearly that loose skin and unequal loss of fat is a temporary state in the course of the diet. Once you attain normal weight, a more equal distribution of your body fat is almost an automatic occurrence. It may take a few months to accomplish, but will naturally result if you are sufficiently motivated to hold your normal weight.

Your face, which may become lean and cadaverous-looking in the course of the diet, will fill out at the expense of slight excesses of body fat elsewhere. In most cases, the loose skin is absorbed. Where the body has passed the age of skin elasticity, a simple surgical operation will remove the excess skin. This is sometimes also necessary in cases of extreme obesity through many years where the skin has stretched beyond the point of being able to shrink to the new conformation of the body.

The reasons which some of your friends may have as the unconscious motivation for their derision of your efforts are unworthy.

Those of your friends who themselves are obese will feel guilty because they have not accomplished the goal you have. They, therefore, will tell you of the futility of your efforts, based probably on their unsuccessful attempts to lose weight.

Some of your thin or normal-weight friends (especially in the case of women) will resent the emergence from the fat-you of a thin-you who will become a rival in their exclusive ranks. Your envious friends, of course, do not experience these emotions consciously. They are able to fully rationalize their attitudes.

Some women patients have found that their husbands are their greatest enemies in the fight to return to the svelte figures of which they once prided themselves. I have found, however, that most husbands are enthusiastic about their wives' dieting. These men fondly hope for the return of the day, just as do the women, when they will be able to show off the slim attractive girl they married. Other husbands display an ambivalent attitude toward their wives—a mixture of love and hate, the latter emotion displaying itself in sadistic treatment.

"My husband has told me how much he is in favor of seeing me lose weight," said one wife tearfully, several weeks after she had gone on her diet. "But he deliberately buys delicacies and things he never did before and eats them in front of me.

"I just love chocolates, French pastry, cream cakes and the like —and he never really cared for them. But now he buys something like that every day and just tantalizes me with them, while he stuffs himself.

"It's been hard enough for me to cope with my own oral desires as it is. Now I have temptation put in front of me almost daily.

"I've told my husband that he has to stop it if he loves me—

and he professes to love me more than ever because of my desire to lose weight. But he thinks the whole thing is a big joke."

There again, the rationalization of these attitudes of sadism which spring up unconsciously in people who ridicule your efforts.

Occasionally husbands have become quite disturbed by their wives' successful efforts at dieting. While they were enthusiastic at the beginning, they become anxious near the end of the diet program when they see their wives nearing success.

"My husband apparently is worried that I may be more attractive to other men, now," said one astute woman who recognized this attitude in her spouse.

"He doesn't really notice it himself, and I don't think he even realizes it, but he uses every excuse he can to get me to stop dieting."

Some husbands have complained that their wives have become too young-looking in comparison to them.

On the whole, however, I have found that most husbands take a deep pride in the success of their wives peeling off excess pounds. They regard it as a personal tribute to themselves and to a successful marriage.

Well-meaning friends will often plague a dieting patient with advice. Discussion of obesity and diets is quite popular in daily life, and somewhat safer than politics and religion. However, this free—and erroneous—advice is quite confusing to many dieters who are paying for professional services from their personal physician. These self-appointed experts utter half-truths with an air of great assurance, but much of the information they hand out is undoubtedly opposed to what the physician has been telling the patient.

You will be told of seven-day diets, twenty-one-day diets, Hollywood diets, and countless other types of faddist diets. Most of these cater to the self-indulgent oral tendencies of the majority of overweight people and for that reason are quite ineffective.

You will be subjected to comparing notes on various books, methods used by physicians, and articles printed in newspapers and magazines. This confusing discussion serves no useful purpose in any sincere weight control program.

You must disregard the advice these well-meaning persons offer and stick with consistency to the program advised by your physician.

The menace of the food faddist is perhaps the greatest of all being given wide circulation today. These faddists have found the field of obesity a lucrative one and they are willing to practice their charlatanism on you with utter disregard of your ultimate health.

They may be well publicized and travel extensively on their lecture tours. They may attract thousands to listen and try—but what they offer is rarely valid scientifically.

Primarily they advise self-treatment. This is potentially dangerous from both the psychological and physical standpoint, even though your best friend may think it's "just the thing" for you.

The thing to remember is to disregard your friends and relatives—unless they tell you to go to a physician and follow his advice. Otherwise you are heading for trouble.

The Fallacy of Fads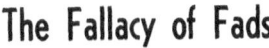

> *The newest fad is the banana-and-coconut*
> *diet. It doesn't help you lose weight, but after two*
> *weeks, you can climb any tree in America.*
>
> DINERS' CLUB MAGAZINE

To SAY THAT WE LIVE in a fad-afflicted country is a mild understatement. Sadly, one of the worst aspects of faddist fetishism in America is the diet for weight reduction.

Diets come and diets go—and the need to diet goes on forever. Why? Because virtually all of the coming and going diets have no lasting—nor often any real—value.

As a more-than-casual observer of the problems of obesity, I have seen diets appear, create a tremendous furor, and then disappear without a ripple. The reason for this is simple. The average person has always looked for a magical answer to his problems— no matter what problems these are or in what area they fall. And, I suppose, he always will—this is the way of human nature.

The natural unconscious wish of every overweight person is to find a formula which will remove the unsightly fat with a minimum of effort and then keep it off in spite of subsequent indulgences in food.

Those who have no knowledge of psychodynamics are amazed

115

at how many intelligent overweight people fall for shoddy gimmicks—gimmicks which cannot stand the light of reasonable investigation. The gullible always have friends who lost an enormous
amount of excess weight by following the principles of the "Blue
Sky Diet" or the book written by "Newblossom Graustark." What
is not fully understood is that there are always people who lose
weight (despite the fact that they soon regain it) and who give
credit to the latest fad diet for their "miraculous" loss. These people
are neurotics who have a strong need to be in the spotlight. They
feel they can, in that way, gain "love," respect and attention. Few
of these people are consciously aware of what they have done.

How true, it now becomes apparent, is the old dictum: "Never
underestimate the power of the unconsious." Equally true is the
fact that if any of these "miracle" diets had the least substance or
validity, they would not have passed out of the public eye and into
medical obscurity. After a few months, the disillusioned—hundreds
of thousands of them—find that they did not truly succeed in losing
weight. And the friend who apparently lost so much weight is now
just as fat as ever. Diet "X" notwithstanding, the friend still wears
a size 20 dress or tips the scales at an ungainly—and unhealthy—
200 plus. For them all, being faddists, the time has come for the
next "miracle diet."

Of course, with the abundance of tempting foods that we have
in this country — and the decline of physical exercise — people
throughout the land are crying out with Hamlet, "O! that this too
too solid flesh would melt." And the lament is answered by innumerable schemes for losing weight quickly. We have passed
through the eighteen-day Hollywood Diet; the banana-and-
skimmed-milk diet; the many diets limited to specific foods that
have been mislabeled "Mayo Diets," consisting, in some cases, of
eggs, in others of rice, or of grapefruit, or even of prunes. Fad diets
so proliferate that an article on dieting in a recent issue of a popular women's magazine could list and describe the *seven* most-
talked-about diets.

116

The Fallacy of Fads

The truly mature individual understands that the problem of overweight is a lifelong problem, a problem that has been successfully coped with by some through careful calorie counting. But he also realizes that the rigors of calorie counting are not practical for nine out of ten obese persons. The difficulty is, how can one always count calories?

The problem of calorie counting was summarized to me one day by a patient. He is a television producer and was, at that time, thirty-six years old. I mention his age simply because he had been dieting, on and off, ever since he was fourteen. He is a well-informed, intelligent man. He was skeptical of all magical claims made by the faddists. Yet he tried to diet in the most impractical way. After unsuccessfully trying calorie-counting methods for more than twenty years, he became a patient of mine and became successful in losing weight and keeping it off.

His comment to me about calorie counting was this:

"You know, Doctor, I've tried one calorie-counting diet after another because that is what practically every doctor advises.

"But the trouble is, how can I measure everything I eat or have my wife do it, or, even worse, have it done for me at a restaurant?

"Worse still, I can't remember all the calorie values of everything. I have many things on my mind, and I can't think of a more unpleasant way to live than to have to carry around a calorie chart or try to remember caloric values.

"Why don't doctors realize that fat people are 'all-or-nothing kids' when it comes to eating?

"To my way of thinking, calorie counting is just as faddist and unscientific as any of the truly fad diets. I feel it's just as naïve as following the advice of those practitioners who say that the only way to lose weight, and to keep it off, is to cut down a little of everything you eat.

"If fat people were capable of following that advice, they wouldn't be fat in the first place."

To which I add—what more can *I* say?

Somebody once said that the worst part of the diet isn't watching your food—it's watching everybody else's. That applies most particularly to the fad diet. How horrible it is to be eating only bananas or coconuts, or rice, or whatever else it happens to be, when everybody else is eating a normal meal. That is why the high-protein, high-vitamin, low-fat, low-carbohydrate diet offered by this book makes life so much easier for the dieter and so much more practical in terms of eating habits and weight reduction.

There are many diets which are nutritionally sound and promise much, yet they are virtually impossible for everyone to follow. The individual personality of the obese person can never be taken into account when devising these "mass market" approaches to dieting. Such diets are obviously created by research and laboratory specialists who do not treat patients or who have only the most superficial contact with overweight people. For some of these creators of diets, the only contact with the obese patient is treatment in a hospital under the most controlled conditions. The controls make weight loss possible.

But such diets get unwarranted publicity outside the hospital —often to the chagrin of the researchers themselves. The Mayo Clinic denies the countless varieties of diet that are passed around from hand to hand in mimeographed form, all labeled "Mayo Diet." There are, officials at the clinic say, countless varieties of diets that are prescribed for patients under their care. But no one diet is meant to be a panacea for all obese persons.

Other diets have been called by names to make them sound authoritative. The so-called Air Force Diet has been denied by every official of the United States Air Force. There was a diet called the Rockefeller Diet which resulted from a controlled experiment at a clinic some years ago. It was not meant, however, for the man on the street.

We should be aware of all the fad diets—in order to be wary of them. What are some of these nonsensical approaches to weight reduction?

A group therapy approach to dieting that has been active in the country for some twenty years is the diet club. This is a mass-membership approach to reducing, and bears such names as "Fatties Anonymous," or TOPS (Take Off Pounds Sensibly).

During recent years, however, something new has been added in the field of diet clubs. This is a purely business operation in which franchises are sold to "successful" members so that they can open and operate clubs in their own communities. Obviously, unsuccessful dieters cannot be given such a franchise because they wouldn't attract members to their club! The new members are recruited by word of mouth and, therefore, the success story of the club leader is the main drawing card.

Is some good accomplished by the diet clubs? To be fair, I must say that some people are successful in losing weight by this means. For the most part these are people who are physically healthy, who are nonpsychotic or only mildly neurotic, and who need praise and social approval to accomplish some unpleasant task such as that of losing weight.

Some of the people who are successful are often most inadequate personalities. They are lonely and frustrated and for them the diet club is the only contact with human warmth. Generally the advice given to people by diet clubs about low-calorie food preparation is excellent.

But there are obvious objections to the diet club.

1. There is no medical examination—only a physical examination—given to new members as a routine and practical matter, although new members are urged to seek medical advice. There are dangers inherent in this nonmedical approach, since members might be diabetic, cardiac or gout patients.

2. The clubs ridicule medication by physicians, and members are told that if they take so-called diet pills they will be dismissed from the club. There is no doubt that such medication as amphetamines has been abused by illegal sources as well as by unscrupulous pharmacists and physicians. But this has also been true in the

119

case of tranquilizers and sedatives. It is dangerous, however, to subscribe to a doctrine of discarding useful medication because of abuses by some persons. Most physicians use these valuable medications with great skill and judgment.

3. It is dangerous to push fragile personalities, such as borderline schizophrenics, to lose weight. The unconscious group pressure in the diet club can result in a highly successful member who was losing weight becoming a full-blown schizophrenic. On the other hand, an alert physician treating such a patient would recognize the appropriate symptoms in such a patient and would take corrective action early. The difficulty is that diet clubs are not equipped with the knowledge of psychodynamics so necessary in the treatment of obesity.

Liquid diets—such as Metrecal, Sego and others—have had a mass vogue for the past few years. These canned foods are vitamin-enriched and of a dairy content. They contain about 300 calories per can.

The sole value to such a diet approach is that the calories are accurately measured for the dieter. An overweight person taking three Metrecal or Sego meals a day will be on a 900-calorie diet and will be sure that the diet contains 900 calories and no more.

Unfortunately, as far as I can determine, there never has been any indication in any of the advertising for these products that the dieter on such a regimen will *not* lose weight *unless no other food is eaten.* Dieters are prone to tell the story about the patient who phoned her doctor to inquire whether Metrecal should be used before or after a meal.

The so-called formula diet, which is designed to help people lose weight by making it unnecessary for them to choose the foods they eat, dates from somewhere in the middle of the last century, when a man named Dr. Philippe Karell conceived the idea of substituting a single food for all the ordinary items in a standard diet, and this fad had a brief whirl. He also used milk as a base for his formula—and milk, or dairy products, have been utilized

120

for this kind of diet ever since.

After Metrecal was introduced to the American market late in 1959, there were many other imitators, including products called Bal-Cal, Quota, and Cloud 900. Though the public has been enthusiastic about these formula diets, doctors and nutritionists have accepted these products with qualifications, issuing warnings to patients about their misuse, and lecturing on the merits of reducing in more nutritive ways.

The formula diet is no panacea for the control of obesity. It should be pointed out that any radical dietary change—such as going onto a formula diet—can be dangerous to people with undiagnosed diabetes, gastrointestinal troubles, liver or kidney disease, anemia, or certain heart conditions such as congestive heart failure.

A highly unsatisfactory approach to dieting, the high polyunsaturated fat diet, was quite the fad a few years ago following publication of a book that sold more than a million copies. Unfortunately, there is absolutely no scientific evidence that eating polyunsaturated fats will cause the reduction of stored fats in the body. Scientifically, the idea of losing fat by eating fat is ridiculous.

The only thing that might happen is that the dieter eventually eats so much fat that he can't stand the taste of fatty foods. He may, therefore, cut down his intake to the point where he could actually lose weight. But if there were any truth in the theory whatsoever, then there would be no problem at all. There would be no overweight people.

There is actually some scientific evidence that the storage of excessive fat in the body will create biochemical conditions which will make it easier for the body to store greater amounts of fat than normal. Polyunsaturated fats, as a substitute in a diet for saturated fats, may lessen the possibility of hardening of the arteries and heart attack—but there is absolutely no relation to weight reduction that can be scientifically proved. The body will store as fat any ingested fats—even polyunsaturated fats—if these fats

121

are over and above the energy requirements of the individual.

The book which propounded this fantastic theory was reviewed by every interested medical periodical. Not one of these knowledgeable medical and scientific reviewers looked upon the theory with favor.

Such a diet tends to reduce weight temporarily through dehydration of body tissue. But nutritionists feel that staying on such a diet for too long can be harmful. It is likely to provide less-than-desirable levels of vitamins (particularly A and C) and minerals (especially calcium). In addition, it has been pointed out that the diet can activate gall bladder disorders and cause other troubles as yet unknown. Persons with diabetes or kidney and liver diseases might also be harmed.

All these objections gain importance in the light of the insistence of the diet's originator that his diet should be followed for life. There is one saving fact: it is highly unlikely that anyone could endure this "dream" diet for much more than a few weeks, to say nothing of a lifetime.

Another book appeared recently with a provocative title that implied that a dieter could drink all the alcohol he or she wanted. This book was soon followed by a series of imitations all based on a low-carbohydrate diet, an imitation of the diet expounded in the book you are now reading.

The authors of all these books claim that the diet is fun to follow (and I am sure that, with enough drinks in one, any diet is fun to follow) and insist that the theory results from an Air Force program which limits the carbohydrate intake of pilots to less than 60 grams daily.

According to this theory, protein is used to rebuild body tissue and carbohydrates and fats are used to supply energy. The authors correctly claim that excess carbohydrate is converted to fat and is stored in the body. They add, erroneously, that since alcohol does not qualify chemically (because it is so simple in structure as compared to complex carbohydrates) it is exempt from the metabolic processes. The truth is just the opposite. Alcohol, being a simple structure molecularly, is more easily converted into fat than the more complex carbohydrates.

Ingested excess fats are the most easily converted into human fats. The manufacturing process in the liver is a relatively simple one—and unit for unit, alcohol will produce more fat than other carbohydrates.

This so-called Drinking Man's Diet is typical of the diet nonsense that periodically sweeps the country. People fall for such a trick diet because it works, for a time, as does any diet in which caloric intake is appreciably less than caloric expense.

This diet, as propounded in one of the booklets that espouse its cause—booklets that had a rapid and phenomenal sale around the country—suggests that "dinner of squab and broccoli with Hollandaise sauce and Château Lafitte, followed by an evening of rapture and champagne with your favorite girl," is the only way to knock off excess pounds. This suggestion probably sounds fine to the girl, but you should be warned that it is not much of a dinner and is not very good nutrition. In fact, it isn't a very filling or satisfying meal; though I must admit that with plenty of champagne and wine the hunger might temporarily be forgotten.

This diet craze is just another adaptation of the old high-fat diet, which has been around for years and which I have already discussed. There are many things wrong with it—as has already been made clear—and over and above that is a fact that the use of alcohol has its hazards. To recommend it deliberately as an important part of the daily food intake for a large segment of the public is poor advice.

Among the many rice diets that have been devised is the Kempner Rice Diet. For many years there has been a trek to the Kempner Clinic in North Carolina as hordes of overweight persons have sought to follow the gospel of losing weight by eating rice exclusively.

There is possibly some value in this diet in the treatment of high

123

blood pressure because it is essentially a low-salt diet. But from the point of view of obesity, it is difficult to envisage any true or permanent value. The diet is dehydrating and sadistically monotonous. In that way, it probably does encourage an apparent weight loss. But, how long does this loss remain with the dieter?

Those obese persons who go to Kempner Clinic live in a somewhat protected environment away from the tensions of their work and their home lives. Therefore they live in an atmosphere that has certain temporary psychological advantages. There is also the comradeship of other people who have a similar problem, and from these people there is a chance of acceptance and approval if successful on the diet. However, back home again, there is no keeping on a rice diet exclusively and there is no maintenance of the reduced weight.

The Hollywood Eighteen-Day Diet is still popular in some parts of the country. In fact, it was once so popular that you could order it in many restaurants. It comprises mainly grapefruit, Melba toast, black coffee, and a nibble of raw vegetable and/or meat.

Another version of the Hollywood Diet was the pineapple and lamb chop diet. This does have some nutritional value and I suppose that, after eating lamb chops and pineapple for a few days, the dieter got so tired of these two foods that the food intake was cut down and some weight was, obviously, lost.

Another area of fad dieting is the starvation diet. In the past two years, there has been some interesting work done by a group of dedicated physicians, working particularly in Pennsylvania and California, who have isolated grossly obese persons in a hospital for a good many weeks and have fed them nothing but water, vitamins and "diet" beverages.

These physicians discovered that after the second day on such a regimen, most of the patients stopped complaining about hunger and then proceeded to lose enormous amounts of weight in what amounted to a crash program. Best of all, the researchers found, the weight reduction was achieved with no apparent ill effects.

These experiments proved, of course, that rapid weight loss for a person who is grossly overweight is both healthy and desirable. This theory has been espoused in this book and was stated many years before these particular, definitive experiments were done.

Unfortunately, practically all the patients involved in these starvation diets proceeded to regain their weight rather rapidly after they were released from the hospital setting. This experience has also been found to be true with patients of physicians who have tried starvation diets privately under similar clinical conditions.

For psychological reasons, I have been dubious about starvation diets as a total treatment process from the beginning—and I have never attempted it with patients even in a hospital setting. It is my belief that the basic oral personality of the obese patient is not changed. Psychotherapy for these obese individuals is most time-consuming and their resistance to such therapy is strong.

I have occasionally used a few days of starvation with patients who proved to be most difficult. But I have always chosen patients who I felt had the intellectual insight into their problem and had the willingness to cope with that problem.

Just as long as Americans abuse the privileges of the plentiful food supply that this country offers and jeopardize their health and fitness by obesity, there is bound to be a mass market for easy ways to weight reduction. However, let it be clearly stated once again: there is no replacement for the intelligent and imaginative control of food intake in proper weight maintenance.

Food fads are undesirable since they may endanger your health. The fads seldom, if ever, have been adequately studied in advance for safety. In addition, to follow a fad almost always means to deviate from a time-tested diet regimen, resulting in little or no benefit.

When talking about the individual who is convinced that some special health benefits will result from the use of unusual food items, I prefer to use the term "food fanatic." It wouldn't be so bad if they kept their counsel to themselves, but they seldom do. They keep on "selling" everyone else on the latest belief—and one fad follows the other.

It is still my belief, and it always will be, that a diet which allows the overweight person to eat without measuring food or counting calories will be most successful in the long run. This is so because such a diet will tend to train them to watch weight more successfully and to teach them to cope with their problem, which is obviously a lifelong one.

The Folklore of Fat ——————————————

Better be dumb than superstitious.

Ben Jonson: ELEGY ON MY MUSE

ARE YOU NOT SUPERSTITIOUS?

Perhaps you don't believe that breaking a mirror will mean seven years' bad luck or some other form of ill fortune. Yet this is probably the most widespread premonition of evil existing today.

Maybe you don't expect anything untoward to happen if you walk under a ladder—again a widely held superstition, one which appears to result from various taboos in many cultures.

There are hundreds of superstitions involving everyday occurrences and commonplace items, as well as customs whose origins are buried in history. The average reader would be surprised to discover the widespread diffusion of superstitious beliefs still existing in every aspect of social life among both the civilized and the savage.

Superstition arises when the mind departs from principles established by experience and reason. It is the irrational fear of that which is unknown, and in time it becomes the folklore, the traditional beliefs, of a people.

127

Many of the beliefs and opinions held by people today are based purely on folklore and superstition rather than on fact. Too often people assume that what they see or hear is "fact," and thus from efforts to explain phenomena and to adapt human activity to the explanations, superstitions arise. It is conceivable that when the scientific method was not known such folklore could become a part of the culture of a people. Enlightenment was further hampered by limited communication facilities, which were such that a truth discovered in one part of the world took as long as decades to become known in another. As science advances, though, superstition recedes. Science brings increasing freedom through comprehension and rational use of natural forces, while superstition holds the human mind in bondage to blind magic and fear.

While the progress of education and the communication of ideas are indicated by the disappearance of superstitions from among the people, it is a surprising thing that so much folklore is still held in wide belief in this day and age. That people today should base belief on observation without reason, on false conclusions due to faulty thinking, or on incomplete obtaining of facts, is incredible.

Among the folklore concerning health and medicine, one finds a vast amount relating to obesity.

The superstitious beliefs surrounding the problem of overweight have become a serious block to many who would embark on a weight control program. They become discouraged at hearing one or other of the tales—stories which in the main are false —concerning the merits of obesity, the perils of dieting, and the misinformation about fattiness.

I am constantly surprised at the stories told by patients whom I would little expect of holding such beliefs. Elsewhere in these pages, some of these fantastic conceptions are discussed in part. I feel, however, that the most common of the false notions should be listed so that they can be controverted here.

From the case histories in my files, I have compiled fifteen of the most common beliefs that patients have used to parry my questions as to why they thought they were overweight.

You may be guilty of believing any one or more of them. That would not surprise me, nor put you in a class by yourself. If you do honestly believe any of the superstitions discussed herein, you have much company. Nevertheless, each of the beliefs I have listed has been uncontrovertibly disproved, thanks to science.

Allow me to disenchant you about your particular pet notion, and to arm you so that you can do battle with those who would dissuade you with beliefs they hold.

Perhaps the commonest misconception is one of which doctors and insurance companies have tried for years to convince the public to the contrary. How often have you heard people say: *"It's healthy to be fat"*?

The very opposite is true: it is unhealthy to be fat! Statistics issued by the Metropolitan Life Insurance Company in 1950 showed that overweight persons exhibit a rate of mortality far in excess of individuals of normal or below-normal weight.

Among the obese, statistics show a greater incidence of high blood pressure, hardening of the arteries, gall bladder diseases and diabetes. The overweight also are poorer risks on the operating table and tend, too, to recover with greater difficulty from, or to succumb to, serious illnesses.

While a great public service has been performed by the Metropolitan Life Insurance Company in their advertisements to instruct the public in the dangers of obesity—among other things—there still is a large section of the population which persists in the false belief that excessive fat not only is harmless, but is healthy.

"Isn't there any other way of my losing weight than dieting, Doctor?" asked a very intelligent woman who was worried about the extra poundage she was carrying. "I've heard of so many cases of people becoming seriously ill due to dieting.

129

"I've even heard of *people who died because of dieting*," she added to cap her argument.

Here is a belief which many persons hold quite seriously. It is based on several factors, mostly stories told by relatives of persons who have succumbed to "wasting diseases." Once the seed of this belief has been planted in the mind of a person, they are apt to find themselves unconsciously associating the wasting effects of tuberculosis and cancer with dieting and resultant weight losing. This is unfortunate!

Dieting to lose excess fat is not starvation. Yet many are the stories which relate that persons actually dying of cancer or some other wasting disease are really on a diet. This is often the case because people tend, unreasonably, to place a sense of shame on cancer and like diseases. They would rather have friends and acquaintances think that dieting is responsible for the loss of weight.

Of course, when the "dieter" dies as the logical outcome of a fatal disease, the legend is perpetuated because of mistaken shame. Much publicity was given recently to the death of a Midwestern socialite. The newspaper obituaries stated that she had died as the result of a strenuous reducing diet. This statement was based on information given to the press by her son. When the facts were made public a few days later, the son retracted his false statement. Unfortunately, as is the case so often with newspaper corrections, the retraction could not receive the same attention as the original story and so went unnoticed by probably ninety per cent of the people who read the original version. The truth was that the woman had died of cancer.

Incidents of this sort have been repeated time and again. Though countrywide newspaper publicity has not always been involved, these false tales have often been allowed to stand and misbelief has spread widely.

There are cases of record where insanity or serious emotional disturbances in which there has been a persistent refusal of food

—such as in anorexia nervosa—have resulted in death. It must be firmly stated, however, that no one has ever become seriously ill through dieting to lose excess fat, when the dieting is done properly and, especially, under the supervision of a physician.

Another widely accepted piece of folklore is that *"body resistance is lowered while dieting."* Persons who believe this will claim that they are more susceptible to colds and other like infections. They will go so far as to blame on their diet a cold which they have contracted in the course of dieting despite the fact that most of the people about them have colds as well.

Even when a patient doesn't blame the diet, friends and relatives often are quick to place the blame and criticize the diet regime. Others will prescribe faddist diets which claim to prevent lowering of body resistance.

This book holds no brief for any faddist diet. As long as the vitamin, mineral and protein intake is adequate, the body will not become deficient in any element necessary for good health. Excess fat is only stored food and the body must utilize it—just as the camel's fat is utilized on long desert journeys—before a person's weight can approach normal.

The obese patient, however, seeks any excuse not to diet. Many of the attitudes concerning weight reduction are based on the natural side-effects of dieting, a matter which is discussed elsewhere in this book.

One man to whom I listed the diet he was to follow and the rate of dieting, came up with another common piece of superstition: *"Isn't it less dangerous to diet slowly?"*

The answer is that it is not dangerous to diet nor is it dangerous to diet quickly. Dieting quickly does not mean starvation. A weight control regime which includes protein foods, vegetables and supplemental vitamins will not permit starvation even though fat is lost rapidly.

People who would prefer to diet slowly are only using this as an unconscious excuse to avoid having to give up the oral satisfactions of eating all the rich and sweet foods they love so well.

A person who is, let us say, seventy pounds overweight, may lose eight pounds during the first week of a sincere weight reduction effort. This is mostly water which stores itself in the fat. Perhaps only twenty-five per cent of the total lost is actual fat, and after a while the same dieting effort will yield only about two pounds in a week. Eventually the loss will drop to about one pound a week.

The amount of fat lost during the regime is practically the same week by week. If, however, the patient fails to maintain his pace of diet, the change in weight loss will be proportionate. Often a patient who will succeed in accomplishing a large loss the first week, will lessen the effort in the flush of success. In effect, however, due to the bulk of water lost in the initial week, the regime will come to a standstill long before the desired weight is reached.

A frequently held piece of misinformation corollary to the last superstition is that *"if weight is lost slowly, you will manage to maintain normal weight much longer."*

Experience has not borne this out. Patients who diet slowly, with difficulty and with complaints of deprivation, will regain more rapidly and will be poor weight watchers. On the other hand, patients who take hold of themselves, throw themselves into a diet regime and lose weight rapidly have shown themselves to be good weight watchers and most of them never regain the weight they took off.

"I'm not nervous when I'm overweight."

This is a belief that may have a vestige of truth in it superficially. One patient who told me this actually felt better when he was overeating. Thus his being overweight was the result of his satisfying oral cravings to cloak many of his disappointments. The fortress of fat in which such persons live will act as a barrier against the onslaught of a "cruel and demanding world."

However, just as a buried, dormant illness is dangerous, so a dormant neurosis is dangerous. It is far better for such persons to reach a state of normal weight and suffer the nervousness which they are cloaking with fat. This is the only way that they have a chance of facing reality and eventually solving their problems in a mature manner.

How often have you heard people say that *"fat people are happy and jolly;* thin people are ill-tempered and unhappy." Fat people then, believe that weight reduction is ill-advised.

Truthfully, fat people act jolly to mask their true feelings. Their reputation for jolliness is undeserved. Obese people are insecure and feel inferior, therefore they are almost unconsciously motivated to be agreeable to associates, relatives and friends.

They feel that the only way they can win love, admiration and respect is by being good-natured and by allowing themselves to become a doormat for anyone who wants to walk over them.

There are many surprises in store for the friends of the successful weight reducer. When corpulent persons attain normal physique, they instinctively show a new willingness to fight for their rights. This, of course, will be used by the persons believing in the superstition of "fat-jolly," to reinforce their belief. They will point to the successful dieter and say: "See how disagreeable he has become now that he has lost weight."

You have but to think a little to recall the number of stout persons you know who are mean, and the number of thin persons who are truly good-natured. This merely emphasizes the complexity of human motivation and reactions and is an example of the possibilities of mixtures and gradations in humans.

"I guess it's just my nature to be fat; it runs in the family."

I see red when I hear this bit of folklore. I cannot emphasize too strongly that fattiness or the tendency to overweight is not inherited.

Physique, body build and stature may be inherited—but not fat. In families where obesity tends to be prevalent, the only reason for this is because of an overemphasis on eating habits.

These usually are families in which rich, starchy and fried foods are served often and in large quantities.

All the emotional factors which create obesity operate in such a household.

Structure of the human body has been divided into three basic types, known as endomorphic, which is the soft rounded type of body; mesomorphic, the hard, square body with well-developed bone and muscle; and ectomorphic, linear, fragile and delicate structure.

These body types refer to body structure and they may be inherited. The fat, however, that may cloak these bodies can be attained in only one way—overeating.

The superstition about glands—*"the reason I'm fat is because of my glands; they're all messed up"*—has been dealt with. Glands may determine the type and distribution of the fat on the body, but they do not create it. Especially do they not create fat in any mysterious fashion out of thin air, as is implied by the frequent claims of portly persons.

Fat is stored food and must be attained from food excesses. These excesses are stored as fatty matter because this is the most economical way in which the body can utilize storage space. Fat is the most concentrated type of food and contains the most calories in the least amount of space.

"Thin people work off their fat in nervous energy, whereas *everything I eat turns into fat and just stays."*

Here is an excuse that is often used. The fallacy here is that only excess food is turned into fat, the normal amount of food needed by the body goes to keep the body in running order. People who claim that everything they eat turns to fat use this as an excuse for their gluttony. It is a feeble excuse, yet I am constantly amazed at the number of sensible people who believe it.

A thin person, as any other person, may work off minute quantities of fat by frequent though purposeless motions, such

134

as constantly shifting in a chair, swinging a leg, tapping a foot, or continuous motion of the arms and hands. But the amount of fat worked off in this way is too little to be of any significance. The truth of the matter is that thin people merely eat less.

A rather unusual bit of belief was sprung on me by a man who said he had been told that *"the best way to lose weight is to eat all you want and work it off in exercise."* This is a great trick if you can do it. For example, if you think of a brisk walk as the type of exercise you prefer, consider that to take off one pound of fat from your body you would have to walk thirty-six miles at a brisk pace all the way.

The energy of one slice of bread would require ten minutes of running to utilize, and a brisk fifteen-minute walk would be required to work off the calories acquired from a teaspoonful of roasted peanuts.

Unfortunately the only thing which exercise will accomplish, aside from tightening up the muscles of your body, is to increase your appetite. In that way the small amount of fat you have lost in exercising is more than made up in the food you will eat to compensate for the increased appetite.

Athletes do, of course, lose many pounds during a contest. This is only temporary, though, and is for the most part water. It is easily regained in the day or two following the strenuous exercise due to an increased demand for water intake by the body.

A great deal of misbelief centers around the fact that *certain foods are not fattening*. The examples given include fruit, nuts, honey and molasses. The fact that all foods are fattening is well established in scientific knowledge, and the foods mentioned here are more so than most others. Among the foods that are more fattening than average, the four mentioned above contain starches, sugars and fats as well as protein. With the starch, sugar and fat content of your diet increased, I need not go into what is going to happen to your waistline in next to no time.

Protein foods, so-called high quality foods, are less fattening

135

because of what is called the "specific dynamic action of protein." But that is something we will discuss later.

Added to the people who have the notion that there are certain glands which can turn air into fat, are the ones who believe that *water turns into fat*. I overheard a conversation in a restaurant not too long ago where one woman admonished a second to cut down on her water intake.

"Excess water turns into fat," she told her with a very knowing air.

This is another good trick if you can accomplish it. Frankly it is as ridiculous as the "air into fat" theory. The body may store excess water temporarily during a weight reduction program and this will result in a "lag period" when weight will hold fairly steady and it will seem as though no fat is coming off the body despite the dieter's great effort.

Actually fat is being lost during this period, but the body seems to retain the water for a while. It must be remembered that during the diet regime your weight will equal the normal you, plus excess fat, plus or minus water. The latter factor in the equation is unimportant. The water is not held by the body for any length of time, and the body can only hold a limited amount of water in any case. When water is held and a lag seems to take place in the reduction program, it will only result in a greater drop in weight in some future week.

The idea, though, that water will turn into fat is baseless. There is absolutely no mechanism in or out of the body capable of doing such a thing.

The "stomach shrinkers" are a peculiar breed who hold a naïve, though understandable, belief that their *stomachs actually become permanently smaller if they should go on a diet*. Many a dieter has found that after a long period of eating less food, he no longer has the desire for or feels the need of as much food as he did and thus becomes easily satisfied with amounts of victuals which would have left him greatly unsatisfied.

Many dieters will attribute this feeling to a "shrinkage of the stomach," a process which does not and cannot occur. The stomach is, after all, only a muscular elastic organ which automatically will accommodate itself to vast changes in the amount of food placed in it.

What probably does occur to the dieter who feels that his stomach has "shrunk" is an actual change of attitude toward food when the realization becomes evident that he is able to function in everyday life more efficiently and stay in better health when he is taking greatly reduced quantities of food. Too, if there is some insight to the emotional mechanisms underlying the tendency to obesity, this attitude is greatly enhanced.

One of the frequent excuses I get from fat persons is truly a complicated piece of what they try to palm off as "scientific reasoning." In the words of a bright young chemist who started to gain weight rapidly after his marriage was annulled, this is what I was told:

"I'm fat because I absorb all the nourishment from my food. Thin people waste their food; most of the nourishment is excreted with the feces."

As this particular patient was a scientist, I was able to refer him to the actual proof in published results of experiment. The proof showed that his theory was completely false.

In the experiment to which I referred him the feces of both thin and fat people were examined for their composition. It revealed that the amount of calories excreted by both types of persons varied so little as to be of no importance.

There are other "tales of woe" and "grandmother's tales" which patients have disclosed to me in confidence or referred to with surprise that I did not know. In every case, the excuse is no more than just that, and in many cases they are too poor to even be considered excuses.

The disturbing thing to me is that some of these stories are told by persons whose intelligence makes the excuse all the more absurd. And while some of the stories are absurd, others verge on the fantastic.

I could go on for pages and pages to list all the childish pieces of folklore and superstition—stories that rank with the belief that spilling salt will mean an argument, or dropping a piece of cutlery will mean a visitor—but it would be pointless. The examples listed here are the most common.

If you seriously think that you know another reason for your obesity—and I can't believe that you do—let your doctor know about it. He will be able to show you the error of your reasoning. We all make mistakes; science, fortunately, can disclose the error and reveal the truth.

"Skinnies" Have Troubles, Too ————————

I am not much in fear of these fat, sleek fellows, but rather of those pale, thin ones.

Plutarch: LIVES (*Caesar*)

YOU HAVE UNDOUBTEDLY ENVIED your thin friends.

Well, before we go any further let me assure you that the underweight person has as much a problem as the overweight.

So often patients have come to me and said:

"I have a friend who 'eats like a horse' and he doesn't gain an ounce!"

It probably is not true; no one can eat like a horse *constantly* and remain thin. But more important from your point of view is the fact that your skinny friend suffers just as much from emotional problems as you.

Underweight and overweight are only the opposite sides of the same coin. Your underweight friend is not a fortunate person who possesses some mysterious factor in his body that prevents any of the "excessive" food he eats from turning into ugly fat.

I have had patients tell me that "life has been unjust."

"Why?" I ask leadingly, and the answer invariably is: "Because I've not been endowed with this wonderful ability to eat all I want and yet not put on extra weight like my friend does."

139

Perhaps it's a wife, or a husband, or a brother—but it's always a "fortunate" person.

Before we go on, let me make it quite plain to you that this attitude will be a serious block in any weight control program you undertake. If you believe that there are people who can eat as much as you and still not gain excessive weight, you are going to feel that dieting is a great and unnecessary hardship. You are going to feel unjustly imposed upon because you have been singled out for such a rigorous task.

There are no people who can eat as much as you and remain lean while you grow fat. There are people who are thin because of serious organic illnesses such as a toxic goiter or Addison's disease, which is a progressively fatal disease due to an adrenal deficiency usually following a tuberculous infection or other chronic infection.

Therefore, there is no need for you to be envious of your skinny friends. Were you to scientifically observe your lean friends for a week, you would have positive proof that overweight is no more than the result of food intake beyond the normal energy needs of your body and that no other factor is involved.

You would notice in such a test several important differences between your own and your skinny friends' behavior.

Thin people tend to overeat only when they are with company. The times at which you have seen your thin friends eat more than you may be the only times at which they eat to excess. Yet you immediately think:

"How can he eat that much and still retain such a slim physique?"

"What you fail to realize," I have always answered patients who ask this, "is that, with your 'skinny' friend, this apparent ability to overeat while still remaining slender is solely an attention-getting device.

"It's of prestige value to him—and he cherishes that value dearly—for it evokes envy from you and others who, like you, overeat excessively. It gives him a certain prestige in your estimation.

"But your 'skinny' friend actually lacks sufficient appetite, for several days following his huge meal in your company, to miss enough meals so that he can make up for his one day's over-indulgence.

"On the other hand, you have probably eaten more than he in the one meal you had together. In addition, you had sufficient appetite to eat a full breakfast the next morning and a couple of hearty meals during that day, and you can keep on that way for days to come without even lessening your usual quota of snacks between meals—fruit, candy and soft drinks which your friend wouldn't think of eating because he doesn't want them or need them."

The body operates much like an engine in that it converts energy. The principle that energy cannot be created or destroyed, but only changed, holds true for our bodies. Energy intake in excess of energy output will accumulate in some form. In the body, the excess intake of energy—too much food—is stored as fat.

For the most part, slim people are completely unconscious of this mechanism within their make-up. They, too, really believe that they can and do eat as much as their overweight friends and are as fully convinced that they don't gain an ounce because they cannot.

Experience has shown that these skinnies are persons who usually hate to eat when alone. Rather than go into a restaurant by themselves, they would skip the meal. Often they will skip several in succession—filling up instead on coffee into which they unconsciously put more sugar than they usually do to compensate for the energy-giving foods they have not eaten.

One of the most difficult cases of weight reduction I had to deal with was the wife of an insurance broker who time after time failed to maintain the gains she had made in her battle with the bathroom scale.

"It's my husband's fault," she finally blurted out to me one day after she prepared to start for the fourth time on a reduction program.

"He eats more than I do, and he doesn't gain an ounce!"

Well, that doesn't make sense. You must realize that as well as I. Yet this woman's charge was no different from many I have heard.

I proceeded to get her to tell me just what proof she had that her husband ate more than she. She stumbled immediately in recounting their breakfasts together. It seems that "hubby" usually only had a hurried cup of coffee and a piece of toast as his day's first repast.

Her breakfast, on the other hand, comprised:

"Orange juice, bacon and an egg—or two eggs—four or five pieces of toast with butter and two cups of coffee."

Quite a substantial start for the day.

A little investigation that night at home resulted in her making the discovery that her husband more often than not forgot—or "didn't have time"—to eat lunch.

I'd rather not say what friend wife ate in contrast to the meager midday meal her breadwinner consumed. Suffice it to say that the lead she took in the morning had by now been well extended. She was winning the race with laps to spare. It was a "walkaway" day after day.

Dinner?

"Well, he eats much more than I do at dinner. He does like his meat extra lean and just loves vegetables. Then he tops this off with a cup of black coffee."

Like Jack Spratt and his wife, the husband's affinity for lean meat was balanced by the wife's liking for the opposite. He could have eaten twice the quantity that she did and still have acquired fewer calories.

Further probing dug up these few telltale facts:

"I don't really eat much between meals—a few pieces of fruit,

142

some nuts, a cookie or two, a bottle of coke, and a few pieces of candy while I watch some of the afternoon television shows."

After the dinner in which her husband "ate much more than I" she admitted to "sometimes two helpings of dessert."

The record speaks for itself. This patient proved more adequately in the telling of her own story what I wanted to prove to her, than I could myself.

What a great many women fail to realize is that if they ate as much as their husbands they would soon approach their weight. For example, if a 125-pound woman ate the identical amounts of everything her 175-pound husband did, she would soon near the 175-pound mark while he wouldn't gain a pound. The food he consumes is utilized by his body to nourish the extra 50 pounds he normally carries. She needs proportionately less than her husband, and so were she to match his eating habits, she would soon become grossly overweight.

In other cases, great differences in the types of food consumed by a fat and thin person will be the key to the latter's "eating more" than the obese member of the duo. Rich, starchy, sweet and fatty foods at the same meal will appeal to the overweight person. The underweight person will, on the other hand, trim all the fat from his meat, eat less bread, spread the butter extremely thin and have an aversion to rich desserts.

These two persons will sit down to the same meal at the same table, yet the overweight person will manage to consume several hundred more calories than the asthenic one. At the end of the meal each will sincerely believe that they ate exactly the same amount of food.

Your underweight friend, then, to repeat, has no magic component in his make-up that makes him someone to be envied. From two standpoints, though, the underweight person has an advantage over his obese friend: (1) he will tend to live longer, and (2) he will have less difficulty with any serious illness he may contract. But as for thinness being something to be envied, no!

143

Asthenia, or underweight, is as much a form of neurosis as is obesity. The exception I mentioned before: the result of an organic illness—which can be demonstrated by clinical findings—such as toxic goiter or Addison's disease.

Many underweight adults were underweight children who refused to eat during their childhood as an expression of hostility to their parents or as a sympathy-getting device.

One mother, for whom I was treating a grossly overweight child, told me of her next-to-youngest who started to "waste away" soon after he ceased being the "baby" of the family.

"Just as soon as my new baby was born, Jimmie stopped eating —almost altogether. He became quite obstinate at mealtimes and we were frantic in our efforts to try to encourage him to take food.

"He just nibbled at a few things, drank some milk, and started to get quite thin. Compared to his playmates, he looked positively ill."

This reaction was a normal one. His parents' concern over his weight and lack of appetite was made to order for his purposes. He had accomplished his aim by diverting attention away from the newborn baby. He reassured himself of his parents' love which they proved again by their concern over his failure to eat.

Even threats and punishment if a child won't eat under these circumstances are evidence to him of their interest in him—and it is such evidence that he needs despite the perversity of such interest and protection.

This attitude then becomes carried over into adult life, especially if the thin-child-now-an-adult has identified other individuals with the roles his parents played in his childhood. Even where the pattern in childhood does not involve sibling jealousy, inattentive or inconsistent parents can be responsible for the creation of a child who does not eat because concern about this will make him the center of attention.

As adults, asthenic individuals are usually overdependent and arouse sentiments of pity in many people because of their thinness and appearance of being weak.

A world-famous crooner, who is often front-page news, was an example of this attitude on the part of the public. Other examples are plentiful! How often have you seen a childlike asthenic, clinging-vine type of woman marry a tall, heavy-set man? How often have you seen marriage between thin scrawny men, and women who are more mature and motherly?

Just as, to overweight persons, obesity is a secondary gain, so, to the underweight, asthenia is a secondary gain. They will unconsciously control their diet to remain thin. They need to stay thin to gain the attention they lack and desire. This dependent role will at times create great interest in their bodily functions. They become prey to many fancies concerning various aches and pains which arouse expressions of sympathy from the person whom they have substituted for the father or mother image. Such persons will often express their need for attention with frequent headaches, palpitations of the heart, or abdominal pains.

One woman's case stands out in my memory. The treatment I prescribed for her was practically identical with that I give to my obese patients, except for diet. It hinged on insight to her problem, followed by a well-balanced high-carbohydrate, high-fat diet in addition to some hormones to encourage her body to retain protein and strengthen bones.

The opportunity to "ventilate" her troubles was the key factor, though, in getting her on the road to recovery. Within a matter of a few months, this childlike-looking woman went from 92 pounds to a normal 116.

Her problem hinged on a sister:

"Ellen is four years older than I (my patient was twenty-eight at the time) and she's always been prettier than I."

That was only the beginning, but from her remark I recognized in what direction the trouble lay and I directed the questioning to bring the nub of the problem to the fore as quickly as possible.

145

"Ellen is quite good-natured," she told me. "She's happily married to an architect who is quite successful. They have three charming children and live in a lovely home in Connecticut.

"I guess it was meant to be that way. Ellen was always more popular than I in our school days.

"Of course, my parents had something to do with that. My father and mother lavished all their love on her because she was so pretty. As a matter of fact, my father, who is retired now, lives with Ellen in Connecticut.

"Not that my parents didn't love me. But as the baby of the family I should have had more love than I got. Isn't it the youngest of the family who always gets showered with love and affection?"

In this case it was the youngest of the family who was jealous —pure and simple.

She is married to a detective on the city police force, a respected though not too highly paying job, and they have one child, a four-year-old son. The resentment she bore her sister for being prettier and hence—in her own illogical "logic"—more loved both by parents and friends of the family, was the unconscious machinery which made her household an unwelcome place to live at times.

Suffering from asthenia, she looked as childlike as she was emotionally. In addition to her thinness, she suffered from severe migraine attacks. When they came—and they lasted for four or five days at a time—they would upset the household to the extent that her sister Ellen would have to come from Connecticut to run things for the husband and child.

In one way this dependence on her sister was an outlet for the frustration she felt at being the "lesser loved" of the family.

After voicing her resentments and jealousies, the younger sister allowed that she felt if she were to gain weight she would be as attractive as her older sister. While much concerned about gaining weight, the woman was a food faddist and a vegetarian. By her own admission she was "a great customer of the health food stores."

146

When she was able to understand intellectually the role which her asthenia played in making her the center of attraction, she quickly responded to the treatment and gained twenty-four pounds in a matter of months.

Interestingly enough, her migraine attacks became minimal in frequency as well as in severity.

The same emotional problems may result in either asthenia or obesity.

Spot Reducing ─────────────────────────

Is this a cause why one should not dine?

Persius: SATIRES

THE BODY'S ABILITY to care for itself has constantly amazed people and probably will ever continue to do so.

Yet, while people slowly come to realize that their bodies can and do adjust themselves, human nature seems to continually trap them into trying artificial aids. Despite the failure of these aids, each new contraption put on the market finds a multitude of buyers. The circle is endless. Successively each gadget is proved a failure; successively each new "invention" is bought and tried.

The problem of removing fat from only certain parts of the body is one which provides the inventors and manufacturers of such gadgets with an endless stream of customers. The manufacturers of these items undoubtedly do a good business because the everlasting wish and hope to attain beauty is one which is strong.

The motivation to become attractive is found in all obese persons—whether they be grossly obese or just moderately so. This motivation is, however, one which is most apparent in middle-aged women who think it fashionable to try to recapture their youthful attractiveness.

In their search for "beauty" these women become the victims of the many commercial gadgets and remedies with which the market is filled—and the claims of which are grossly untrue.

To put it simply—and perhaps disappointingly to many—there is no such thing as spot reducing.

There are many reasons why a person may develop excess fat or flesh in any part or parts of the body. Unfortunately these persons usually become quite gullible and develop into avid purchasers of mechanical devices in their attempts to reduce large hips, heavy thighs, pendulous abdomens or other enlarged parts of the body. Their efforts in this direction are always unsuccessful. None the less they are never deterred, it seems, and they continue to try new devices and new "cures"—to the monetary benefit of the manufacturers of such.

There are many glandular disorders which favor the formation of "fat pads" in certain regions of the body. As has been stated earlier, there are no glands which create fat; but glands will determine the distribution of fat on the body.

The only hope of remedy is in general weight reduction. Where such a program does not result in the correction of so-called figure faults—after a period of time—there is no panacea to accomplish the desired result.

Hormones or gland substances which might be used in the treatment of these "illnesses" offer little hope at this time, as current knowledge and available weapons to treat these conditions are limited. Endocrinology as a medical specialty has made great strides in the past quarter-century but the answers to many perplexing problems still have to be obtained from discoveries yet to be made in that field.

Among the more common "spot fat" illnesses are:

Cushing's disease which results in enlargement of the trunk of the body, and the face becoming "moon shaped."

149

The hypogonadal woman with deficiency of ovarian hormones who will have heavy hips and upper thighs.

The hypothyroid or myxedematous patient who will develop a fat pad on the nape of the neck.

The aged or hypogonadal male who will find himself with abdominal fat deposits while retaining relatively slender arms and legs.

The Froelich type of obesity in which there is excessive fat on the middle part of the thighs, and in the girdle area.

Progressive lipodystrophy where there is gross obesity of the lower half of the body while the upper half becomes emaciated.

Added to sufferers from these illnesses are the patients whose difficulties with spot reducing are caused by the underlying bone structure and not the muscles and fat which cloak the bones. Women with a wide pelvic girdle, bowing of the upper thighs and thick wrists and ankles can never truly hope to remedy these natural structural "faults." Many of these hereditary traits are desirable from the point of view of strength, good health and ease in childbearing—yet they do not conform with the ideals of feminine beauty in our Western civilization.

Women who are built thusly should accept these attributes with full recognition of their advantages. They must also accept the fact that if they do not fit into society's concept of feminine "beauty," it cannot be helped in any way. They must not think of themselves as "deformed," "misfits," or "ugly." They are merely the result of heredity, much the same as every other person.

It is possible that unusual builds—by our standards of beauty—are the result of dissimilar body types in parents and grand-parents. A woman whose ancestors on her paternal side were tall and slender with delicate bone structure, and on her maternal side were short, stocky, muscular and large-boned, may inherit an incongruous combination. She may have a small face with slender arms and small breasts and then flare to large hips, heavy thighs and oversized ankles. A woman so built who tries to utilize every way possible to make the lower part of her body attractive to match the upper part will find the results unsuccessful and probably agonizing.

An opposite type of body is possible—and has occurred. In these instances you will find large faces, heavy shoulders and a large abdomen set on incongruously slender legs. The efforts of these people in spot reducing are just as fruitless and heartbreaking.

Many are the men, approaching middle years, who notice with dismay that their abdomens have become larger than desirable. Some perhaps remember their youth: days on the beach when they were bronzed demigods in their bathing suits. They feel that they have been putting on weight and ought to reduce. They have not necessarily been gaining weight, for the relaxing of the abdominal muscles which occurs as an almost natural process with advancing age, results in the internal abdominal viscera and muscles relaxing and "falling," giving the appearance of fat. This is known as visceroptosis and is a quite common occurrence.

The unsightliness of a relaxed abdominal wall is, of course, aggravated by layers of fat over unused muscle. This obesity may be corrected by proper dieting and the relaxed abdominal wall may be improved temporarily by exercise. Where visceroptosis is extreme it becomes a medical necessity for the patient to utilize an abdominal support.

It is no disgrace for a man to wear a girdle. Unfortunately too many men who would be benefited by abdominal supports and girdles are reluctant to utilize these valuable aids. They are motivated by a fear of criticism. They are afraid they will be ridiculed by their friends.

Women, on the other hand, have utilized the girdle to great advantage to support their relaxed abdomens. This perhaps is the reason men shy away from girdles. They feel that these aids have been identified in the public mind as a purely feminine contrivance. There is no reason why this should be so. The girdle is no more an aid for women than are eyeglasses, hearing aids, orthopedic shoes or any such. Men have the same trouble with slackening viscera as do women and should make available to themselves the same aids.

Exercise, as has been pointed out, may temporarily aid relaxed stomach muscles. But exercise is not practical for most middle-aged persons. Magazines and newspapers have reported many varieties of exercise designed to remedy figure faults. The average reader, however, does not realize that a complete change in a way of life is being suggested to him.

To assume glibly that a few weeks of intensive exercise—or fifteen minutes every day—will greatly change the contour of the body is naïve. All patrons of "slenderizing" salons or eager exercisers for short periods have discovered that failure to continue the exercising or treatments indefinitely means a return of the muscle laxness.

The amount of exercise advisable for a young person whose occupation is sedentary, or the middle-aged person, is perhaps eighteen holes of golf once a week and an occasional long walk.

Modern man who no longer lives in a hunting-and-fishing-for-a-livelihood culture, as did his ancestors of thousands of years ago, is not conditioned to vigorous exercise beyond the days of his youth. Vigorous exercise for most persons is not healthful or desirable because it may put persistent demands on the heart and circulatory system beyond their capacity. Real damage can result.

The narcissistic desire to create a "body beautiful" may destroy a person before his allotted years. A healthy and attractive body is a worthwhile goal, but the man of forty-five who wants to look like a college athlete is foolish indeed to train as seriously and as hard as the youth twenty-five years his junior whom he is trying to emulate.

There have been exceptional persons, of course, who have gone into their later years with the muscular bodies of youth. Most of us are less fortunately endowed. We would be placing a strain on the body far beyond its capacity were we to follow their example.

The vogue of massage, both for spot reduction and general weight losing, has become quite popular with the fashionable middle-aged woman. Not only is this a useless procedure, it is potentially quite harmful.

Most people are dismayed at the prospect of the sacrifices necessary in a diet regime. Additionally they are horrified at the prospect of exercise. The appeal of massage, then, is great. Here, they think, is a treatment in which all that is required of them is to lie down and allow someone else to do the work of taking off excess pounds.

It is highly questionable whether so-called massage will break up fat pockets. And, contrary to popular opinion, massage will not cause the absorption of loose skin. It will cause loose skin to become looser still because the effect of massage is to break down subcutaneous connective tissues. The skin thus loses its support—just as if you were to take the ribbing out of a dirigible balloon —and hence becomes even looser.

Heavy massage is especially undesirable because the tissues may become bruised. In the case of massage to legs which have varicose veins, injury to the veins may be caused with resulting thrombophlebitis. In some cases a secondary infection of the limbs may develop with a fever of long duration and the releasing of blood clots into the general blood stream.

Light massage of any part of the body is indicated only where impaired circulation requires such treatment.

Mechanical devices on the market generally utilize the massage principle or passive agitation of the muscles. The same objections which apply to massage and exercise are congruous to these gadgets.

The use of Turkish or steam baths merely involves the principle of encouraging perspiration. The loss of sodium chloride and water due to the profuse sweating will result in a temporary drop of weight. However, as soon as the resulting thirst is satisfied, the weight will return to its former level.

Practical spot reduction is possible, but only where there is general weight reduction to a normal level first. When the desired level is reached and held for a few months, fat on undesirable locations will be redistributed by the normal processes of the body.

Frequently patients who have achieved their desired weight level find themselves perhaps with drawn faces and a padding of fat on some other part of the body—the hips, the stomach. If they continue to stay at their normal weight, they find that within a few months the face will fill out and the fat pad disappear.

A redistribution of body fat seems to occur for most people after a successful general weight reduction regime if the weight is held at the normal level for a reasonable length of time. It must be made clear, of course, that this is possible only if the underlying general bone structure is normal. A large pelvis or bowing of the upper thighs cannot be corrected.

The fat over a relaxed abdomen can be removed by dieting. The flaccid abdominal muscles and the bulging of the abdominal viscera cannot be helped by dieting alone.

If you have passed the age where exercise will help a relaxed abdomen, let your vanity allow you to wear a support, not prevent you from doing so.

THE SOLUTION

Principles of Weight Reduction _____

All people are made alike.
They are made of bones, flesh and dinners.
Only the dinners are different.

Gertrude Louise Cheney: PEOPLE

UNLESS YOU CAN ACHIEVE some understanding of the basic emotional problem which has resulted in your obesity, you cannot have ultimate success in any weight reduction program.

If you have tried to lose weight before and have failed, it has been because you did not realize that your problem is emotional. Now that you know of the emotional basis of your overweight, you can achieve the necessary insight. This insight need only be superficial—that is, intellectual as opposed to emotional—to help you control the symptom of obesity.

Weight reduction in most cases is an important therapy involving principally cooperation between the patient and the physician. The treatment combines both psychological and medical aspects. Practically all physicians have the knowledge and resources to deal with such cases, though many have been offhand with the average obese patient.

Few obesity patients require major psychotherapy or depth analysis. Those who do have many psychological stigmata in addition to their obesity. They are resistant to minor psycho-

157

therapy and medical treatment. Such patients have to be referred to a psychiatrist for the intensive therapy necessary for treatment, for in such cases obesity is merely one symptom among others which point to a major psychological difficulty.

Such persons require true emotional insight before they can go about helping themselves in regard to any of their symptoms, including obesity. True emotional insight is difficult to attain. It requires years of intensive psychoanalysis in many cases.

Many intelligent, well-read patients accumulate the jargon of psychoanalysis and believe that they truly understand their problems. It is, however, not that easy. It is one thing to say "I have an Oedipus complex," or "I have a feeling of inferiority," and another to feel oneself into the exact emotional connotation of these situations.

For example, were you to tell a person to imagine that his home is burning, he could contemplate the situation calmly. That is intellectual feeling. Tell him to imagine that the house is crumbling on his children, their clothes are afire and they are crying piteously. The difference of his attitude gives the clue in the difference between intellectual and emotional insight.

There are rare cases of obese persons who have dieted on their own and successfully remained at normal weight. These cases are as rare as self-cures in other serious diseases.

The vast majority of obese persons require all the help they can get in solving their problem. Especially do they require help in initiating the program of weight reduction.

Too often persons who would never attempt to indulge in self-medication if they were suffering from arthritis or heart disease are just the persons who will attempt self-treatment for obesity. They do this, little realizing that obesity also is a serious illness.

Many such persons are quite intelligent, yet they will follow superficial advice on dieting they read in newspapers and magazines. Or they will listen avidly to the strange ideas of friends.

Any individual strongly enough motivated in seeking weight

reduction will lose weight on practically any diet. Once the motivation is removed, however, the pounds will go right back on again.

An example of this is the young woman about to be married. Some months before the wedding she will go to her doctor to get a diet so that she will slim down to agreeable svelteness. Generally, she should be successful in reaching her goal and holding her weight until the nuptial date.

Such persons are quite willing to give up their oral drives for a while in order to accomplish some temporary goal—in the above instance, the woman wants to be a beautiful bride. Soon after the "goal date" has passed, the pounds go on again because the motivation has passed, too. The wedding and the honeymoon are over and the obesity reasserts itself.

For complete success, insight and understanding—*not merely motivation*—are necessary.

The role of the physician is paramount in any weight reduction therapy. Physicians find that practically all patients interested in losing weight know all about which foods are the most fattening and which are the least fattening. The average obesity patient usually has accumulated an amazing amount of knowledge regarding diets and calories. The physician in most cases has little instruction to give the patient regarding diet, other than to straighten out misconceptions.

The failure of any reducing diet is never the lack of knowledge. Any reducing diet favored by the physician will be successful if all other factors are attended to as well.

Your physician's attitude toward you will be most important in the treatment.

As a practitioner, your doctor undoubtedly likes people, or else he would have gone into some form of practice where he would not have been dealing with people, but would have been able to put his scientific knowledge to good use in such things as pathology and research.

Do not think that because you are obese that you are considered by your physician as "second rate," that you are despised consciously or unconsciously and merely dismissed with advice to eat less.

Doctors realize full well that all humans, including themselves, have emotional difficulties in some area of their lives. Therefore, you will find that your doctor will have understanding of your difficulties no matter what they are.

It is, of course, far easier for a doctor to treat a case of acute appendicitis. Treatment involves only the removal of the offending organ. Within a week, the doctor has a cured and grateful patient. But the physician treating obesity is prepared to curb all feelings of impatience he may develop with a patient who will unconsciously resent the doctor for having deprived him of the pleasures of eating.

The physician is prepared to expect a series of bizarre symptoms from his obesity patients—most of which are purely unconscious protests against dieting. The physician is ready to curb himself from criticism and sarcasm when the patient starts to criticize the physician's methods—for the obesity patient will use any excuse to rationalize his avoiding continuance of treatment.

Some patients will tell their physician: "I don't feel well in some ways, therefore this dieting must be bad for me." And this is an attitude that even the most intelligent patients who fully realize the dangers of obesity will use.

Your physician will insist on a rigid schedule with regular visits. His role in your reducing is that of the authority to whom you must report regularly. Your understanding of this fact is paramount in the psychotherapy of obesity. Once you realize that you must report regularly to your physician, you will undoubtedly attempt to make as good an effort as possible for each visit.

Similarly, you will find that your physician will not neglect the medical aspect of weight reduction. He will treat you as a complete individual. As a patient for obesity you are going to be more time-consuming to your physician than his other patients. But your physician will not deny you time whenever you want to "ventilate" your emotional difficulties. Your physician realizes that this is the most important aspect in the therapy.

Few obesity patients are masochistic enough to be browbeaten into dieting, and so your physician will display the utmost patience with you, rather than display any anger he may feel at your sometime halfhearted efforts.

Many obesity patients, as has been pointed out, will utilize anything as an excuse to stop their diet regime. Relapses are understood, and your physician probably will calmly discuss the reasons for your relapse with you so that you will understand them and attempt to make up for the setbacks in the weeks that follow.

The role you as the patient play in a weight reduction regime should be one in which an attempt is made to understand the drives to overeat. You must not attempt to evade or rationalize the responsibility for your obesity. You cannot blame your obesity on glands, heredity or any factor outside your own responsibility.

You must realize that dieting without understanding of the basic motivation behind overeating will never be permanently successful for the average person. The pleasures of overeating will not be given up by a patient, for instance, who lives a relatively empty, routine, boring life. Here overeating will have to be supplanted by some other interest. Therefore, rely on your physician's advice and help. After all, he has been trained to help you. He will do no harm to you, despite some of the "strange symptoms" you may suddenly think you have developed during dieting.

Diets involving special menus, calorie counting and portion measuring have proved themselves impractical in most cases. The weight reduction diet advised in this book is a healthy diet. But it should not be undertaken without the guidance of a

161

physician who will advise the use of those supplemental vitamins he thinks necessary in your particular case.

The basic idea of any diet, however, is simplicity. The average person is not mathematically or scientifically enough inclined to be able to follow the diets ordinarily advocated in reducing.

When it comes to food, you must consider yourself much like the alcoholic with liquor. Just as the alcoholic should not be trusted with the first drink, so the obese patient should not be trusted with starches, sugar and fats during a diet regime.

After you have reached your goal and have acquired a degree of insight, you will be able to go on a more liberal diet during your weight-watching period so that you do not lose more weight than necessary. This, however, will be discussed in full detail in a later chapter.

The basic reducing diet recommended is high in protein and low in starch, sugar and fat.

Water and salt are not restricted. This is unnecessary in practically all reducing regimes and is potentially dangerous in some cases. Salt restriction may be essential in cases of cardiac failure or high blood pressure. But it is never necessary for dieters unless there are these medical indications as well as obesity. Your physician will decide this matter for you.

Thyroid medication also is unnecessary—except in the relatively rare cases of myxedema which has been discussed earlier. Thyroid prescribed in obesity may result in a depression of normal thyroid activity and thus create a dependency on the hormone. The increase in metabolic activity by thyroid pills is never enough to accomplish any appreciable weight loss, unless the patient also diets. In that case, weight loss is the result of the dieting and not of the thyroid medication.

Hunger-curbing tablets have been found valuable in a weight reduction program. But if the patient indulges in self-medication with such tablets, the treatment may become pernicious and useless after a while. Any regime which relies solely on such medication along with diet, and pays no attention to psychotherapy, is sure to fail after many relapses.

During the period when the obese patient must not only deprive himself of guttony but must eat less than normal-weight individuals, hunger-curbing tablets are of great help. The patient requires all the help he can get at this time. After the patient attains normal weight, he will be able, with his own resources, to keep his weight down.

Above all, it is well to remember that hunger-curbers are not particularly toxic or dangerous compared with other common medications used for other diseases.

The difference between success and failure, however, in a weight reduction program is psychotherapy and the resulting understanding the patient attains of his problem.

No amount of knowledge of the calorie content of all foods and the principles of good nutrition will enable a patient to diet, to persist in dieting, and to be able to remain at normal weight the rest of his life.

So-called "common sense" advice—"use your will power," "do it for a couple of months and it will be easy after that," or "you ought to be ashamed to be so fat, especially when it is so dangerous"—will not motivate an obese patient sufficiently to persist in losing weight and staying normal.

Diet's the Thing ───────────────────────

Touch not; taste not...

COLOSSIANS 2:21

OVERWEIGHT IS ONE CONDITION that can be prevented or corrected.

If you are overweight, it is only because you overeat. Therefore, there is no other way for you to lose weight than by eating less.

There is a proverb in French which says that appetite comes with eating. But so does obesity.

Obese people may attempt to reduce, but the emotional cause of their overeating remains to trip them up. Appeals to their vanity rarely help. Showing them the health hazards of overweight does little good.

Therefore, insight of the factors which create your desires to overeat must be acquired so that you can have the proper motivation to diet, so that you will be able to stick to your diet, and so that you will be able to remain slim after diet has brought you to normal weight.

You now understand that there are cases where overeating may be caused by a desire to build a fortress of fat, or cases

164

where it may provide a secondary gain, or others where it may be due to childhood patterns of oral eroticism.

Knowledge of these facts provides the insight which in turn gives you the drive to diet. But knowledge alone is not enough. You must diet in order to attain normal weight.

Medical authorities have advocated many methods of dieting. Any of these will prove successful to a patient strongly enough motivated to diet or to one who has insight to the emotional problems which cause overeating.

Nutritionists have created high-protein diets, low-protein diets, egg diets, banana diets, vegetable diets, and fluid diets, among others.

Most of these, however, have become outmoded with increasing knowledge of all the factors—physical and emotional—which cause obesity. The recent diets used in reducing programs all demand calorie counting, and from this a new variety of diet has been created: the 800-calorie diet, the 1,000-calorie diet, the 1,200-calorie diet, and so forth, depending on age, sex, occupation, and the amount of weight to be lost.

This is all very well, desirable and scientific. It probably is the ideal way in which weight should be lost. But it is not practical for most obese patients.

The typical obese individual will not count calories, measure portions nor religiously observe for more than a few weeks at a time the complicated regime necessary for this method. Recognition of this fact is shown by the calorie-counting gadgets so common today. One of the most clever is a series of daily menus with attached tabs on which are printed the various items and their caloric content. As you eat each item listed on the menu, you destroy the corresponding tab. At the end of the day, the "bank" may contain 50 or 100 calories which have not been used in the daily allowance. These calories are applicable to the next day's allowance.

Another convenient calorie counter is a scale on which all

common foods are listed with their equivalents. Thus when confronted with a restaurant menu, the obese person merely refers to his counter and figures out his permissible indulgences for that meal. Some restaurants now print caloric values on their menu items.

While some of these methods are tedious and others are not, all encourage the tendency to do a little cheating on the diet. Forbidden sweets are attractive and the obese patient rationalizes that he will make up the overindulgence the next day.

This is much like the alcoholic who rationalizes each drink as "only one more," or perhaps says that he will stop after "only one drink." The diet cheat is no different from the man "on the wagon" who after passing all the bars en route home after work, turns back to the last one for one drink as a reward for having passed by all the bars.

Just as the alcoholic must not be indulged in a "first drink," so the dieter must not be indulged during a weight reduction regime.

The type of diet advised by the author is one which requires the supervision of a physician. The diet, along with the other principles involved in the weight reduction regime used here, has proved successful for many patients. If all the other factors required are attended to, then the diet is the vital factor in successfully losing weight.

While some doctors may firmly believe in calorie counting as the correct way to diet, this is a method that works for only some people. I have found that most patients have great difficulty adhering to a calorie diet, while they have followed the diet recommended here most successfully.

The diet I recommend is one which can be followed more easily by the patient during the weight reduction regime and results in successful removal of excess weight. It exemplifies, too, the principle that an obese patient's overwhelming desire for oral satisfaction in sweet and rich foods should not be catered to.

Two principles are required in following the diet:

1. With the exception of eggs, foods which are permissible may be eaten in unlimited quantities and as often as desired.

2. Foods which are not permissible may not be eaten at any time.

In other words, quantity of permissible foods on the diet is not curbed by any means. You may eat all you want of the foods permitted.

In this circumstance you can never complain of not having had enough to eat—you can fill up.

The diet may be called an "exclusively high-protein, low-carbohydrate and no-fat" diet. It permits great quantities of foods high in vitamin and nutritive content and generally forbids foods low in these qualities.

Practically all foods rich in vitamins, amino acids (the "end" products of protein digestion) and minerals are allowed.

Foods rich in easily available calories are forbidden. Obese persons have a great number of calories stored in their excess fat and weight cannot be rid from the body unless these calories are used up. The principle, then, is to utilize the calories already stored in the body for energy.

The patient is permitted all the lean meats, poultry and seafoods desired. But all the visible fat must be trimmed from these foods.

Fried foods are absolutely not allowed.

All but five vegetables are allowed. These—the most common of the starchy vegetables—are potatoes, corn, peas, rice and beans of all types except string beans.

This concept allows for a healthy menu with many variations.

While dieting to lose weight, the patient is allowed no sweets, starches or fats of any type. In keeping with this rule, the following common foods are forbidden:

Bread, butter and fat products, cereals, fruits (with certain exceptions) and soups (except meat bouillon).

The average obese patient will exclaim on seeing this diet: "What, no fruits? not even a little ice cream? not even the smallest piece of cake occasionally?"

The answer is a simple No.

The reason for this answer is that practically all obese persons are like alcoholics. I call them "victualics." Permit them an occasional sweet or starchy dainty, and they will almost invariably take more.

It is easier to adhere to a strict simple diet. In this way there is no possibility of cheating.

If the patient cheats, he is likely to find at the end of the week that he has lost few or no pounds. His morale is broken because he has already overestimated the sacrifices he has made. This he will utilize as an excuse not to diet any longer.

The temporary lack of success leads again but to excess.

"After all," the patient rationalizes, "I've done practically everything my doctor told me to, and nothing has happened. It must be due to my glands, at that."

A number of patients when told of the diet they have to follow have all but cried to me that they would "starve." This is ridiculous. The quantity of lean meat, poultry and seafood, as well as of the permissible vegetables, is not curbed in any way. Therefore there is plenty of food to fill the void.

Another question frequently asked is: "Where will I obtain the energy calories necessary for me to function?"

These are supplied by your own body. The fat body contains countless calories taken from food indulged in in the past and stored in the most economical way nature can—as fat.

Even though fat is sharply curtailed in the diet, adequate Vitamins A and D are obtained from eggs, which are permitted in a limited number (one a day in my basic diet), and from yellow vegetables. It must also be remembered that even the leanest of meats has some fat in it, despite what the patient will trim off.

The fruits and vegetables permitted in the diet provide adequate quantities of Vitamin C. The unlimited quantities of protein foods permitted provide a superabundant amount of B-complex vitamins and minerals.

Supplemental vitamins are given, regardless, as a margin for safety. This, however, is something for the physician to give advice about, as each individual case is different.

Most physicians will want to prescribe one of the many hunger-curbing medications now available to make the dieter's task easier.

Salt and water are not restricted in the diet, for if there is any danger to dieting it will be because of such restriction and not because of the rapid weight loss.

The patient next thinks of another problem...

"Do I have to live on a diet like this all my life?"

The answer is that sacrifices are to be expected in curbing the oral demands no matter what the weight reduction regime is. Once normal weight is attained, however, the patient can eat as much as any other individual of a similar constitution and still hold his weight. While losing several pounds a week entails some sacrifice, staying at normal weight does not.

The principal difference between persons of normal weight and those who are obese is that the former regulate their food intake unconsciously and the latter must regulate it consciously. The conscious regulation is not truly sacrifice.

Certain points of the basic diet herein prescribed will be further elaborated and explained in chapters which deal with specific dynamic action of proteins, water balance, vitamins, hunger-curbing medications, and side effects.

You will note that the basic diet calls for small breakfasts. I do not believe in the idea of large breakfasts which have been advocated by some nutrition experts. Their claim is that a large breakfast "will start the day off right" for the dieter who then will be able to adhere to a calorie diet for the rest of the day and thus lose weight.

Their theory is that the large breakfast enables the dieter to acquire the necessary energy to cope with the day's problems. This advice, in my opinion, ranks equal with that of eating a piece of candy before a meal so that the sugar in it will take the edge off the appetite, thus making the patient eat less at his regular meals.

My personal experience with obese patients is that if they eat a large breakfast, they will not deny themselves large lunches or dinners.

In fact, I have had some patients, including those of normal weight and some underweight, tell me that a large breakfast only seems to increase their appetites during the day, while a small breakfast acts conversely. It seems that most people can function quite adequately on, and prefer, a small breakfast.

Rare is the obese patient who objects to a small breakfast on his diet. The obese patient's true eating problem comes later in the day and in the evening when snacks between meals have been usual.

The trouble with too many weight-losing diets is that they have been drawn up on the theory that the patient will fall in with the ideas of the expert. Instead, the diet has to be practical. It has to fit in with people's actual eating habits.

That is the basis upon which this diet has been conceived. That is the plan upon which the basic menu presented here is based.

It has been my experience that giving the widest possible consideration to a patient's eating habits in prescribing a diet menu has been by far the most practical method of aiding the patient in following a reducing diet.

With the number of foods permissible there are many palatable variations of the basic meals given here. Knowing what you may and may not eat makes it possible to utilize this basic menu in conjunction with any diet menu given by nutritionists. The basic meal listed for lunch and dinner may be interchanged as necessary.

THE BASIC DIET

Breakfast
a half grapefruit
(or a small orange)
an egg (boiled)
one slice of protein bread (if desired)
coffee, tea or skim milk

Lunch
vegetable juice
(four ounces)
lean meat or pot cheese
large salad
coffee, tea or skim milk

Dinner
bouillon
lean meat, fowl or seafood
one green and one yellow vegetable
one - quarter melon (in season)
or tomato juice (four ounces)

The salad suggested for lunch may consist of any of the permissible vegetables, but it should be remembered that oil and mayonnaise dressing are prohibited. Vinegar or lemon juice with a touch of salt and pepper makes a very tasty dressing for salad and brings out the natural flavor of the vegetables.

Tinned and frozen foods are packed under scientific control by the most modern of methods. They are wholesome, sanitary, thoroughly cooked and easily digestible. They retain their vitamin and mineral content to a high degree.

Moderation should be exercised in the intake of vegetables in a raw state. If eaten raw in excessive amounts they may prove irritating. It is advisable to balance your vegetable intake by having at least half of those you eat cooked.

Seafoods which are wholesome when eaten alone do not become poisonous by admixture with other foods such as milk. Poisoning or injury from food combinations is unknown.

Now that you are ready to diet, here is a list of rules which are vital in your weight reduction regime. Study them carefully and obey them. There are multiple purposes for each. Failure to abide by any one of these rules will set up the first pitfall to failure in your diet.

A DOZEN DOs AND DON'Ts OF DIET

1. You MAY eat all the lean meat, fowl and seafood you want. *Nothing may be fried and all visible fat must be trimmed off.*
2. You MAY NOT eat bread or butter. *While a slice of protein bread is permissible at breakfast, it should be omitted if possible.*
3. You MAY NOT eat peas, corn, rice, potatoes and beans (excepting string beans). *Other vegetables are allowed in unlimited quantities.*
4. You MAY NOT eat fruit, *excepting half-grapefruit or an orange at breakfast and melon for dinner dessert.*
5. You MAY NOT eat sugars, fats or starches.
6. You MAY NOT eat breakfast cereals.
7. You MAY NOT eat soup, *except clear bouillon.*
8. You MAY NOT drink fruit juices, *but vegetable juices are allowed.*
9. You MAY NOT drink liquor or soft drinks. *Where business obligations may require you to take liquor, two drinks are the maximum and may be taken only straight, with water or soda.* COCKTAILS ARE OUT, *but tea and coffee may be had in unlimited quantities (with skim milk and artificial sweetening agents).*
10. You MAY use all condiments. *Neither salt—*NOR WATER*—need*

be limited, except when your physician finds a medical indication to limit these.

11. You MAY NOT use oil or mayonnaise, *but ketchup and cocktail sauce may be used sparingly and lemon juice or vinegar may be used as wanted. (Mineral oil should* NEVER *be used as this coats the intestinal wall and prevents absorption of vitamins.)*

12. You MAY eat snacks between meals. *These should consist of tomatoes, cucumber, raw carrots, celery and lean meat*—IN ANY QUANTITY DESIRED.

At first glance, the diet prescribed may look meager. It is not, for not only is there a wide variety of foods that are permissible, but you can eat as much of these permitted foods as you want. Here are planned meals for seven days which show how complete and interesting a variety of menus can be prepared:

FIRST DAY

Breakfast

one-half grapefruit
one boiled egg
one slice of protein bread
coffee

Lunch

tomato juice
grilled lean hamburger
celery and radishes
tea

Dinner

shrimps with cocktail sauce
roast leg of lamb
Brussels sprouts and cucumber salad
coffee

SECOND DAY

Breakfast

one sliced orange
one slice of protein toast
coffee

Lunch

tomato and lettuce salad
broiled halibut
spinach and boiled carrots
skim milk

Dinner

mixed vegetable juice
lean corned beef and cabbage
melon
coffee

THIRD DAY

Breakfast

one-eighth honeydew melon
one poached egg
coffee

Lunch

bouillon
tomato stuffed with crab meat
tea

Dinner

carrot sticks
steak
turnips and string beans
coffee

Fourth Day

Breakfast one-half grapefruit
one slice of protein bread
coffee

Lunch carrot juice
salmon and chopped onion salad
celery and radishes
skim milk

Dinner bouillon
broiled calf's liver
mushrooms and broccoli
coffee

Fifth Day

Breakfast one-quarter cantaloupe
one boiled egg
coffee

Lunch bouillon
fresh vegetable salad
cottage cheese
tea

Dinner tomato juice
roast veal
squash and beets
coffee

Sixth Day

Breakfast
quartered orange
one slice of protein toast
coffee

Lunch
tomato and lettuce salad
two hard-boiled eggs, carrots
skim milk

Dinner
mixed vegetable juice
swordfish steak
asparagus tips and cauliflower
coffee

Seventh Day

Breakfast
one-half grapefruit
one poached egg
coffee

Lunch
bouillon
broiled lamb chop
stewed tomato and green pepper
tea

Dinner
celery stalks
roast chicken
endive and kohlrabi
melon
coffee

Eating Out _____

There is no love sincerer than the love for food.

George Bernard Shaw: MAN AND SUPERMAN

"THERE'S ONLY ONE SMALL DIFFICULTY," say a good many patients after we've discussed the diet they are to follow until they successfully reach their desired weight.

"And that is 'eating out,'" I add, knowing well what to expect.

Many people have to contend with eating restaurant meals due to business commitments; others have certain social obligations that have to be fulfilled during the diet regime. Whatever the reason, many patients seem to feel that if they eat a meal in a restaurant they are going to be forced to break the diet plan.

This is absolutely not so.

You can eat in any good restaurant, choose from the regular menu, and still follow the diet prescribed herein with little or no difficulty.

Good restaurants prepare each dish individually. In this way, right at the start, you have only to tell the waiter that you are on a no-fat, low-carbohydrate diet, and he—and the chef—will give you the utmost cooperation.

Even if your commitments take you to a French restaurant,

an Italian restaurant or a kosher Jewish restaurant—where food is served traditionally rich—you can with a great deal of facility order foods which are principally high in protein and which are prepared in a fashion that will keep you strictly on your diet.

To prove this point to the satisfaction of my patients, I spent some time talking to the chefs, headwaiters and managers of a number of New York's leading restaurants. All expressed a great deal of interest in the diet as well as in the treatment I prescribe. Some already were acquainted with the diet, having catered to some of my patients on various occasions. In no case did I find a restaurant unable to serve a number of dishes which would conform with the diet.

Pat Moriarty, the owner of P. J. Moriarty's Chop Houses, who has had wide restaurant experience, made it a point to state that in any restaurant the waiter should be instructed to have a dish prepared without dressing or butter.

"As long as the dieter explains what he wants," he said, "we'll go out of our way to see that the instructions are followed to the letter."

In a steak house you will encounter no difficulty whatsoever. Most do their meats over an open flame without any fripperies. All you have to do is cut off the visible fat, or order it cut away.

At Moriarty's the excess fat on every piece of meat is trimmed before it reaches the fire. The remaining fat is easily disposed of after the meat is done.

A typical meal at Moriarty's might be:

melon
roast sirloin of beef
tossed salad
string beans and stewed tomatoes
coffee

That's a huge meal, enough to satisfy the hungriest person and yet fully within the confines of the diet. Among alternate choices to be had for the main course are broiled chopped sirloin steak—

served here in huge portions—or two other specialties of the house: calf's liver steak with onions and broiled club steak.

At Rattazzi's, one of New York's most famous Italian restaurants, owner Dick Rattazzi pointed out that among the high-protein foods on every day's menu will be found chicken Riganata —prepared with parsley, vinegar, garlic and oregano; broiled flatted veal cutlet served with lemon; and broiled shrimps with lemon sauce, to name but a few.

The usual Italian dishes with pasta or parmigiana are out, of course. Yet there remain many other dishes from which to choose. For example, you might order:

pickled mushrooms

consommé

scaloppine of veal all'agro

zucchini and escarole

melon

espresso

Seafood, of course, ranks well up on the high protein diet scale. Oysters, clams and lobster are available in many forms and are quite as delicious served without butter sauce.

"Many people don't realize how good fish is when it is steamed," said Adolph Flashner, owner of The King of the Sea restaurant. "Actually, a piece of fish steamed and then seasoned with lemon juice and salt is extremely delicious and highly nutritious."

A typical seafood meal might comprise:

shrimp cocktail

clam broth

steamed sea bass

carrots and string beans

coffee

The regular cocktail sauce may be used with the shrimp. Lemon or salt, or both, will bring out the flavor of the bass.

There are many alternative choices that may be had in a sea-food house. Among the appetizers are lobster cocktail, crab meat cocktail, oysters or clams with cocktail sauce, or clam juice. Clear green turtle soup may substitute for clam broth. Lobster can be served broiled or steamed. There are many fish that can be used for the main course, or finnan haddie can be ordered, or even a cold seafood platter, without dressing.

The problem of serving a meal sans sauce, something not normal in the French cuisine, didn't cause Lawrence Romano, owner of Laurent's, to bat an eyelid. He admitted that, as in an Italian restaurant, there are many dishes that have to be avoided altogether to meet the dictates of the diet.

"But there is much that a person can order and still not feel out of place or that by dieting they are missing out," said our host.

"It is important to tell the waiter that there must be no fat or sauce," he reminded, echoing the words of everyone who discussed eating out and following a diet. Among the dishes recommended were smoked beef tongue, frogs' legs, duck, and lamb steak. A typical meal might consist of:

madrilene
broiled sweetbreads
endive and braised celery
demitasse

The Chinese restaurant offers much variety to the person on the diet. Jimmy Lee, manager of Lum Fong, made it a point to note that many dishes prepared in the Chinese fashion are sautéed in strained chicken broth, rather than in butter. Mr. Lee also pointed out that in dishes where a flour binder is required, the Chinese chef grinds his own water-chestnut flour, with extremely low starch value, for this purpose.

Dishes recommended in the poultry category included Moo Goo Gai Pan, Chow Sang Gai Pan, and chicken with tomato and green pepper. Other main courses could consist of a combination plate of Chinese vegetables; pepper steak; bean sprouts and shrimp; and Choy Sum Ha Kew, which is shrimps with hearts of bark choy and Chinese vegetables.

For a meal, you might order:

water cress soup with beef
Ngow Yook Kew
(steak and mushrooms, Chinese style)
tea

What about the kosher Jewish restaurant? Here again we encounter a kitchen where food generally may be expected to be prepared richly. This I discussed with Lou G. Siegel, who runs an establishment which bears his name. He also emphasized that the waiter should be told of the no-fat, low-carbohydrate diet so that he can help you select to avoid sauces and rich dishes.

I learned that a specialty such as gefüllte fish is prepared without bread crumbs or matzo flour. Thus it is a perfectly acceptable delicacy to order when prepared in this fashion: three types of fish mixed with a little egg which acts as a binder.

Other typical dishes include roast spring lamb, roast veal, roast fowl, prime ribs of beef, and steaks and chops off the grill. An average meal might be:

sliced calf's brains
boiled beef flanken
fresh vegetable salad
melon
tea

The argument that the patient cannot maintain social engagements and still continue on the diet to the letter of the rule proves baseless.

The Stuff of Life _____

To eat is human, to digest divine.

Charles T. Copeland

"WHY DOES MY DIET have to consist mainly of proteins?"
"What exactly is a protein?"

Ninety per cent of patients ask these questions. They are
especially common from patients who have been on diets before.

To most persons who have attempted to reduce—and to other
overweight individuals who have contemplated the idea but never
done anything about it—the principle of diet has seemed to be
calorie counting.

This is all very scientific. The only difficulty is that to follow
a calorie diet to the finest degree you would have to carry a
complete chart of foods with the caloric value for each, and a
scale to weigh every portion you eat, and you would have to
make the effort to find out fully what went into the preparation
of everything you consume.

"An impossible task, isn't it?" has been the rejoinder of the
average person to whom I have explained this.

I'd say, "It's more than impossible."

To get back to the diet, then, let us find out just what protein

183

is. All the food you eat is essentially one of three types: fat, carbohydrate and protein.

Basically, protein is the *stuff of life*.

"Stuff of life," that's a catch phrase—meaningful but perhaps meaningless without a basic knowledge of what part protein plays in your system. By "stuff of life" I mean that it is the primary part of all organs and tissues in all animals and plants. It is the only truly living portion of any tissue.

Protein is an extremely complex matter. So complex, in fact, that by contrast starches, sugars and fats—which serve the function of nourishing tissue or acting as reserve material—are infinitely simple in their structure.

To the question why the diet prescribed must consist principally of protein, I have a simple answer:

"Let us reduce protein into terms with which you are more familiar—calories.

"Proteins proportionately have the lowest calorie content of the food types. Therefore without having to work mathematical miracles and juggle complicated figures, you are eating the foods which can supply only the lowest possible caloric content.

"Without a superabundance of calories, and the added fact that the food you eat is pure tissue builder, your body has the least chance to absorb fat from your meals. The body, therefore, must utilize the stored fat, or energy, and the result is a wearing away of your excess pounds."

I have found that most patients receive this information with a great deal of interest. Many even inquire as to the actual process of digestion and metabolism and they claim it has helped them to clarify most of the misconceptions they have regarding obesity.

First, digestion is the breaking down of food into component substances. Metabolism, consequently, is the building up of these substances into living matter.

In digestion, basically what happens is that substances manufactured by the body, called enzymes, attack the food you eat.

These enzymes are catalysts which bring about a chemical change in the food by breaking it down to simpler substances so that the system can start to utilize what it needs where it is needed.

"You have to look at the process like that of building construction," I explain. "Building materials have first to be created out of trees and rocks and raw metals. In the body the equivalents are proteins, carbohydrates and fats.

"The protein enters the body in large chunks, and these get broken down to smaller parts which are called amino acids. The carbohydrates, in order to be used in the building, are broken down into sugars, or glucose. The fats are split up into glycerine and other substances known as fatty acids.

"Now you have all the material necessary for the building. These are the foundation materials for metabolism. But you don't start building your house where you made lumber from the trees, or shaped the rocks into building stones, or refined and molded your metal.

"These substances therefore are absorbed into the system for transportation for where they are needed in the building process.

"Inside your system, the amino acids and sugars get into the blood capillaries and are dispatched all over the body to feed the cells.

"The bogeyman of the digestive process is the product of fat digestion. It is a slowly moving bunch of tiny fat globules which have recombined after digestion and move about the body in what is known as the lymphatic system.

"While the blood carries the other products to their jobs quickly, the lymph—a fluid similar to blood plasma which fills the spaces between the tissue cells—acts like the stagnant water in a swamp. It has little or no movement.

"What immediately happens, then, becomes obvious, does it not?" I ask at this point.

"Of course," the patient replies. "The fat sort of gets congested around the body."

185

"Exactly. Fatty deposits are laid down in various parts of the body, usually in layers under the skin or in more remote recesses."

There are two phases of metabolism—a building up, called anabolism, and a breaking down, known as catabolism. Within certain limitations these processes will allow amino acids to be converted into glucose (if needed) and thence into fatty acids which are in turn built up into fat. Conversely they will allow stored fat to be converted into fatty acids and then into glucose.

Digestion and metabolism are processes which, like every other activity of the body, require a usage—or loss—of energy. This energy usage in these two particular processes is called the Specific Dynamic Action (SDA) of foods.

The SDA of protein is far in excess of that of starches, fats and sugars. This is due to the complexity of proteins which require that the great organ of metabolism, the liver, expend much energy in breaking down amino acids. It has also been postulated that amino acids exert a direct influence on cell metabolism and cause the oxidation of fats, sugars and starches to take place with more vigor.

Because of the great SDA of protein, as well as the quality of its essential factors to living tissue, high-protein foods have become extremely popular in all reducing diets. Any diet high in protein will be rich in all essential amino acids, vitamins and minerals. In this fashion the body is fed all the essentials except the fatty acids so that the fat-storage areas are required to give up their fat little by little to feed needed quantities into the system. Additionally, a high protein diet is palatable to most individuals and tends to satisfy most hunger.

As the body's tissues comprise largely protein, it is obvious that only the protein part of food can supply that material which is required for the replacement of tissues used in everyday wear and tear on the body. Fats, starches and sugars cannot be built up into protein because they do not contain one essential of a protein—nitrogen, which is necessary for maintenance and growth.

All classes of food which contain protein may be utilized as "fuels" for the body. Another unique aspect of proteins is the fact that they supply the body with a substance the body is unable to synthesize, that is, make itself. This is a chemical combination, known as a "ring" grouping, which is indispensable for the manufacture of essential hormones and enzymes.

The liver plays a great part in metabolism and is primarily responsible for the large SDA of protein, for, to do its share, the liver expends much energy.

The liver continuously manufactures bile—which is stored in the gall bladder—for intermittent delivery to the intestine to aid in the digestion of fat. The bile salts hold the fatty acid in solution to facilitate its absorption.

Fatty foods which are metabolized by the liver into glucose are utilized in one of two fashions: either to fill the energy requirements of the cells; or turned into fat and stored in the "fat depots" of the body for later usage. Thus when the amount of food ingested is greater than the requirements of the body, the result is overweight. Because the cells are being fed all the energy they require, the balance of the food is turned into fat for storage.

Another role played by the liver is to remove the nitrogen from the amino acids. The nitrogen, utilized partially as ammonia for the body to neutralize the metabolism's acid end-products, is non-combustible and therefore is not needed in the action of giving energy.

The liver splits off the nitrogen in the form of ammonia in a process known as deamination. This is a fundamental reaction in body chemistry. The remaining molecule is a carbohydrate containing carbon, oxygen and hydrogen—all combustible and therefore able to act as fuel and supply energy.

While the ammonia's uses are primarily in neutralizing acid, the liver may also take intermediary products of the deamination and build them up to glycogen, glucose, or even fat for storage. This is not a simple process, however, and does not occur easily due to the complexity of the amino acids.

The SDA of protein involved in these actions of the liver can consume as much as thirty per cent of the total protein ingested. It is obvious, then, that protein as a food "wastes" a large portion of itself in energy used for conversion. And as certain amino acids can never be converted into glucose and thence to fat, due to the complexity of the structure, proteins give little or no fat to the body for storage.

On the other hand, the SDA energy requirements of fat, starches and sugars, is only about five per cent. With so small a loss in the conversion of these carbohydrates, due to their relatively simple structures, they are easily converted to glucose by the liver and then go through the other metabolic steps to become fat and attach themselves to the fat-storage "depots" in the body.

So it is that a diet rich in protein and low in starch, fat and sugar will force the body to utilize its stored fat for everyday energy requirements. An obese person with a great deal of excess fat stored in his body will immediately have the fat deposits utilized to supplement the high-protein diet prescribed herein.

It was believed at one time that a diet low in starch, fat and sugar would produce during metabolism an organic compound known as ketones. These ketone bodies must be oxidized by the tissues. But when they are produced too quickly for such a "balancing" action there is a potential danger to the body, because the blood's acid content becomes greatly increased. Experiments and clinical observations have proved, however, that this viewpoint overlooks one important factor. That is that obese people have sufficient stored fat for all the energy requirements of the body and do not develop ketosis—an excess of ketone bodies—during a weight reduction regime.

Uncontrolled ketosis occurs when ultra-thin persons are starved. In such instances the body's protein—not the ingested protein—

is being utilized for energy and is being broken down. Ketosis also occurs in uncontrolled diabetes, but due to another mechanism which it is unnecessary to describe here. Ketosis cannot occur in obese individuals because the liver converts the stored fat into glucose easily.

Amino acids, one of the essentials of the SDA of protein, are among the simplest building blocks of protein metabolism. They are essential for life and for the well-being of the individual. They fall into two groups. One group is essential for building tissues. The body cannot produce these particular amino acids; they must be supplied in food. The second group is not essential to life. Their purpose is primarily to supply energy. If these are not available in the ingested food, the tissues can synthesize some of them.

Animal proteins—lean meat, poultry and seafood—are usually first-class proteins and contain all the essential amino acids. Vegetable proteins are considered second-class as they contain only a few of the essential amino acids.

Ill effects have never been known to follow a high-protein diet. Lower forms of animal life have been shown to live in good health indefinitely on a diet exclusively of lean meat. Eskimos, who live in a hunting and fishing culture, exist on an almost exclusively meat and fish diet. They do also consume large quantities of fat in order not to lose weight, but the lack of starches and sugars in their diet has proved entirely unharmful to their well-being.

Devising a reducing diet requires thorough utilization of all these factors.

It has been estimated that a manual laborer with an energy output of 4,000 calories a day would, on a strictly meat diet, have to eat eleven pounds of lean meat daily to balance this spending force and thus keep from losing weight. Since such a diet is not feasible, this person can use larger quantities of starch, sugar and fat. A person of sedentary habits actually requires almost as much protein as a person at hard labor, but far less carbohydrates and fat.

A diet, therefore, must be devised with the idea that it is desirable for the obese person to lose weight. The diet should make this possible for him. Too many diets have been created on the premise that the patient is of normal weight. These are "maintenance" diets, calling for foods to keep a balance in the body and requiring normal poitions of carbohydrates and fat.

In a reducing diet all the factors discussed here must be taken into consideration. It should therefore call for a great deal of lean meat, poultry and seafood, and be low in fat, sugar and starch.

Of course, it is understood that even the leanest of meats have some fat in them. As much as carbohydrates are avoided in the diet, more than enough will be supplied regardless. The body's fat will be adequately broken down, ketosis will be prevented, and the goal of weight loss reached.

Medication

The physician is superfluous among the healthy.

Tacitus: DIALOGUS DE ORATORIBUS

OUT OF PRACTICAL CONSIDERATIONS the obese patient needs a "crutch" during the sacrifices of a weight reduction regime. For this reason many physicians have found hunger-curbing medication—anorexients—of great value in the treatment of obesity.

Before discussing these so-called "reducing tablets," let me make two points clear.

1. The "patent medicine" kind you can buy in any drugstore are generally of no value.

2. Hunger-curbing medication has been incriminated as the cause of many "dire consequences" in the current folklore of obesity.

The medicines sold openly in drugstores without a prescription are generally useless. There are many brands on the market, but most of them consist of "sweets," or vitamins and do not contain any of the medication employed in the regular anorexients. This, in the public's interest, is regulated by the Federal Food, Drug, and Cosmetic Act.

The theory behind the "sweet" content of these medicines is

191

that if sweets are eaten before meals, the appetite will be cut down. Other of these medicines contain vitamins on the basis that vitamins are given in a physician's treatment. But the physician prescribes vitamins as a safeguard against a deficiency during the dieting, not as a magic method of melting off fat or a nostrum to curb hunger. Vitamins can do neither of these things.

If the naïve purchasers of these patent medicines were to read the "fine print" of the advertising both in publications and on the packages, they would find that they were being slightly misled into believing that the medicines will do all the things they give the impression of doing.

There are also patent medicines which involve the use of cathartics. They, too, are useless in the therapy of obesity. In addition, they are potentially dangerous if taken in the presence of a serious abdominal illness.

Many misconceptions have grown up in the public's mind regarding anorexients—some possibly because of the patent-medicine type of treatment. A number of these misconceptions have, however, developed due to normal *side effects* which any drug or medicine may have.

Be assured that most of these medications have little or no harmful side effects when utilized by physicians.

All of the "wonder" drugs, hormones and antibiotics now in use have side effects and may cause complaints. These depend upon the "sensitivity" of the patient and the dosage necessary to treat the illness involved.

In diseases such as arthritis, drugs are used which have many potent side effects. Therapeutic weapons such as gold salts and cortisone must be used with caution by physicians, yet their great value has been clearly demonstrated.

There is little adverse comment about this type of medication in the treatment of arthritis, but the amount of criticism of anorexient medication in the treatment of obesity is unduly great. The criticisms come mainly from lay sources. They are, in fact, based on the emotional context of the obesity problem. The criticisms are not valid.

Since the advent of amphetamine sulfate, or Benzedrine, on the market years ago, there have been many improvements in this type of therapy.

Probably the oldest modern medication used in the treatment of obesity is thyroid extract. This was utilized in the belief that obesity was a glandular disorder involving an insufficient production of hormones by the thyroid gland. This is only true in the relatively rare cases of myxedematous obesity, the aspects of which have been discussed earlier in this book. It is known that one of the functions of the thyroid is to speed up the rate of the metabolism. In all cases of obesity, except for myxedema, the rate of metabolism is normal. A speed-up is undesirable and unnecessary in treatment. Overdose of thyroid will cause palpitations of the heart and may put a great deal of strain on the circulatory system.

Thyroid has never been found effective in reducing. It is used only in cases where a marked thyroid deficiency is noted in the patient. It is well to note that even in clear-cut cases of myxedema, dieting is necessary—as well as thyroid therapy—to attain normal weight.

The use of other hormones or gland preparations, such as pituitrin, female hormone and male hormone, have been tried in the past without success as far as obesity treatment is concerned.

Digitalis, belladonna, iodine and barium compounds were tried with little success in the past. In the light of present-day knowledge, these drugs are greatly outmoded and no longer utilized.

Bulk laxatives are used by some physicians on the theory that rapid excretion of digested food may prevent complete absorption, and that the sense of fullness in the intestinal tract will assuage a feeling of hunger.

Probably the most common ingredient in the bulk laxatives is

193

methyl cellulose. This is a hydrophilic colloid and remains liquid in the stomach and small intestine. It forms a smooth gel in the colon and is supposed not to cause distension and bloating of the abdomen.

A recent addition to the list of bulk laxatives is wafers which contain 1.5 grams of methylcellulose in a wheat flour base with sugar, salt and other flavoring added. Each wafer is the equivalent of 30 calories. While these wafers are probably at best merely an adjunct to other methods of therapy in selective cases, it is not possible to evaluate their effect as yet.

The most valuable medication used in the treatment of obesity is the anorexients. In addition to curbing the feeling of hunger for most patients, they also impart a sense of well-being, or euphoria. This additional property is valuable because obese persons feel that dieting is a great sacrifice. They require elevation of the mood in order to improve morale.

Hunger-curbers have been proved effective in laboratory experiments with animals, such as rats, which eat considerably less when given the medication. This is proof that the medication has an organic effect on the body and is not used merely for the benefit of "suggesting" that it will have an effect.

In discussing anorexients the difference between hunger and appetite must be clearly understood. There is often confusion regarding these terms; people fail to distinguish between them. Hunger is the physical craving for nourishment. It is a basic animal drive which humans share with the other members of the animal kingdom. In addition to hunger, however, humans with their particular psychological make-up have developed appetite—an oral sensation which may persist after hunger has been satisfied.

Appetite is the feeling experienced by people who have already eaten a complete meal and still desire some such item as a sweet dessert to satisfy their taste sensation.

No one has ever seen an obese wild animal. The animal has a

194

hunger drive which is satisfied by eating. The animal doesn't think of food again until it gets another hunger drive. The animal's hunger is teamed with its food needs. Humans, on the other hand, remember the taste of a certain food and go back for more. And they remember the pleasant associations of eating—whether it is to ease an anxiety, to achieve a secondary gain, to fulfill a social function, or any of the other aspects we discussed earlier in this book.

Anorexients have their greatest effect on hunger. They have little effect on the sensation of appetite. Patients rarely complain, however, of either hunger or appetite while using hunger-curbing medication.

The great evil of hunger-curbing medication is that of self-treatment. All therapy with medication of any type should be under the supervision of a physician, trained to understand the properties and dosages of all drugs. Too many dieters unwisely obtain a supply of this type of medication and either use it improperly so that the advantages obtainable are lost, or attempt to overdose in order to make up for overindulgence in food—a ridiculous theory.

The belief that overdosage of anorexients will make up for food overindulgences is based on the false idea that these medications actually take weight off and that dieting is therefore unnecessary. This is, of course, not true. Hunger-curbing drugs merely curb hunger sensations and elevate the mood. They do not melt fat away magically.

Perhaps the best-known hunger-curbing medication is Benzedrine. It is used in psychogenic depressive states and is effective in controlling hunger. The makers of Benzedrine and Dexedrine —also a hunger-depressor —state that they should not be used in patients hypersensitive to ephedrine. Nor should they be used in agitated pre-psychotic states or in cases of coronary heart disease.

Dexedrine sulfate, or dextro-amphetamine sulfate, has fewer side effects than Benzedrine and is used in depressive states, obesity control and other widely dissimilar conditions such as alcoholism and the nausea and vomiting of pregnancy. A new form of Dexedrine has become available, called Dexedrine Spansules, a "sustained uniform release capsule." When used to control appetite in weight reduction, Dexedrine Spansules maintain a constant braking effect on hunger. Only one capsule a day is necessary. The same precautions which apply to Benzedrine apply to Dexedrine.

Another medication is a combination of Dexedrine and Amobarbital, a mild sedative. It is used to relieve depression, anxiety and tension and for those overweight individuals who are overstimulated by the amphetamine family of drugs.

There are many other amphetamine medications on the market, put out by various reputable drug manufacturers under various names. They are similar in action depending on the combinations and dosage.

Many dieters are acquainted with the multicolored tablets which generally contain amphetamine, phenobarbital, thyroid, atropine and a cathartic in various combinations and used in various dosages. Most of the ingredients are unnecessary and potentially harmful if used over long periods. It is well known that many patients use these tablets without supervision of a physician and for long periods. This practice is to be condemned.

Artificial sweetening agents, such as saccharin and Sucaryl, are extensively used by dieters. These substances contain no calories and are therefore freely used in place of sugar which does contain calories. They have been proven to be perfectly safe to use over long periods.

Why Vitamins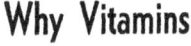

The belly will not listen to advice.

Seneca: EPISTULAE AD LUCILIUM

"BUT VITAMINS IMPROVE the appetite and put weight on a person," patients confront me with regularly. "Why have I to take them if I'm dieting?"

That is a common misconception which is understandably gathered from the most common usage of vitamins. Vitamins merely prevent or cure illnesses caused by vitamin deficiencies. In most cases persons suffering in this way are emaciated. Their cure entails putting weight on them while building up the vitamin content of their bodies. If the vitamins given to these persons improve their appetites, it merely shows that a vitamin deficiency state has been aided.

Vitamins will not, however, improve the appetite of an obese individual—especially during a diet regime.

Their inclusion in the reducing program is merely to prevent the possibility of a vitamin deficiency illness, for at times a patient will not follow rigidly the diet prescribed. These patients are inclined to color their statements as to how closely they are following the advised diet. Therefore, while not necessary for most

197

patients, supplemental vitamins—as well as minerals—are given to avoid trouble.

In effect, they add an ounce of prevention while pounds of fat are being melted off.

What is a vitamin?

It is one of a group of seventeen known organic compounds found in variable, minute quantities in natural foodstuffs. They are required for the normal growth and maintenance of the body. They cannot be created by the body and therefore must be obtained from outside sources.

Since everything you eat is balanced for vitamin and mineral content, as well as for protein and low fat content, let us examine the vitamins.

Vitamin A (axerophthol) is formed in the body from the yellow pigments of most vegetables, called carotene. It is essential to create new cell growth. It aids in maintaining resistance to infection and it delays senility.

In excesses it may cause bone fragility, drying of skin, enlargement of the liver, loss of hair and a morbid state of the blood.

Deficiency of this vitamin can result from inadequate intake, or can result from diseases of the abdomen—celiac diseases and sprue. A lack of the vitamin may cause night blindness—nyctalopia. It may also cause conjunctivitis and xerophthalmia, diseases of the eyes. A lack can also be responsible for dry, rough skin and papular eruptions of the skin. There can be impairment of bone and tooth formations. A proneness to infection and general debility are also possible.

Among the best sources of vitamin A are: asparagus, beet greens, broccoli, carrots, eggs, liver, spinach, fish and fish-liver oils, and tomatoes.

It is well to note that the use of mineral oil may cause poor absorption of vitamin A.

There are many members of the vitamin B group. Vitamin B_1 (thiamine) is essential for normal digestion as it improves the tone of the gastrointestinal tract. It also is necessary for growth and the normal functioning of nerve tissue.

A deficiency of this vitamin can cause an impaired carbohydrate metabolism and beriberi (common among peoples whose diet is limited to such foods as polished rice). There can be damage to the heart, with enlargement and cardiac failure, and damage to nerve fibers.

Among the better dietary sources of vitamin B_1 are wheat germ, milk and various meats.

Vitamin B_2 (riboflavin) acts as an enzyme in cellular oxidation and reduction. A deficiency may cause cataracts, dimness of vision and abnormal pigmentation of the iris. It may also cause a scaly skin condition and cheilosis, which is lesions at the corners of the mouth. Retardation of wound healing is another result of a deficiency of vitamin B_2.

The best sources of this vitamin are: eggs, kale, liver, milk and turnip greens.

Another important member of the B group is niacin. If deficient, the principal result is pellagra, a disease characterized by diarrhea, dermatitis and dementia (often called the "Three-D disease"). Along with a deficiency of niacin, there must be a poor protein diet if pellagra is to develop.

The dermatitis of pellagra resembles sunburn in the early stages. This is followed by nausea, vomiting and watery stools. Depression, impairment of memory and dementia follow in the later stages.

The best dietary sources of niacin are: beef, chicken, fish (especially canned tuna) and liver.

Vitamin B_6 (pyridoxine) is essential for the complete metabolism of tryptophane—one of the principal amino acids of protein, a deficiency of which aids in contracting pellagra. B_6 also is associated with the metabolism of the essential unsaturated fatty acids.

A deficiency may cause a dermatitis and anemia.

199

Principal sources are beef liver, cabbage, chicken, halibut, loin of pork, turnips and wheat germ.

Another fragment of the B-complex vitamin is pantothenic acid, which is essential for all living things. The exact role it plays in humans still is the subject of much controversy, but it is apparently related to the utilization of other vitamins.

The main sources are beef heart, beef liver, broccoli, cauliflower, eggs, mushrooms and wheat germ.

Three more of the Bs are inositol, choline and folic acid, all found in quantity in meat, poultry and fish.

Inositol is concerned with the metabolism of fat and cholesterol.

Choline improves the transport of fatty acids from the liver to the fat depots. It is utilized in treating fatty livers and various cirrhoses.

Folic acid is used in the treatment of pernicious anemia and is essential for the metabolism of growing tissues and cells.

Vitamin B_{12} is needed for the treatment of pernicious anemia, as well, and for sprue. In children, it is a growth factor.

Milk, meats and egg yolk are the principal sources.

Vitamin C (ascorbic acid) is important for bone formation and repair, tooth formation and wound healing. It is associated with the metabolism of certain amino acids.

A deficiency causes scurvy, which is characterized by swollen, tender joints, loose teeth, weakness and hemorrhage in various parts of the body. A delayed healing of wounds also is prevalent.

The best sources of vitamin C are: broccoli, Brussels sprouts, cabbage, kale, lemons, mustard greens, green pepper, spinach and turnip greens.

Vitamin D is formed of the ultraviolet irradiation of foods. It increases the absorption of calcium from the intestinal tract and aids in regulating the calcium level in the blood.

An excess amount of this vitamin will mobilize the phosphorus and calcium from the body's tissues and may cause symptoms of nausea, headaches and weakness.

A deficiency of vitamin D will affect chiefly the bones and teeth. It is the cause of rickets in childhood and osteomalacia (bone softening) in adults. Retarded growth and lack of vigor are common symptoms of such a vitamin lack.

Good sources of vitamin D are: eggs, herring, liver, mackerel, salmon, tuna, milk and fish-liver oils.

Vitamin E (tocopherol) is found in a wide variety of foods and is necessary for normal reproduction in many species of the animal world. Its significance for humans is still highly controversial. It is regarded as an antioxidant which preserves easily oxidized vitamins and fatty acids in foods and in the body.

Good sources are: steak, liver, celery, eggs, turnip greens and fish-liver oils.

Vitamin K (phylloquinone), essential for blood clotting, is isolated from green leaves in its natural form, but can be produced synthetically. It is used to combat bleeding diseases. In deficient quantities it can cause multiple hemorrhages in subcutaneous tissue, the bladder, kidneys or brain.

Normally it is available in cabbage, cauliflower and spinach in the greatest quantities.

It is important to note that vitamins will not cause increased appetite in a weight reduction regime in spite of popular superstition. Vitamins merely prevent a vitamin deficiency illness. Patients with a vitamin deficiency illness will have improved appetite when this lack is supplied. People who have an adequate amount of vitamins in their diet will not acquire an increased appetite when taking vitamins.

Minerals and Elements _____

'Tis not the food but the content...

Robert Herrick: CONTENT NOT CATES

"YOU MENTIONED MINERALS being given to prevent trouble during a diet regime. Just what minerals are they? I know that, for instance, ordinary table salt is made of sodium and chlorine. But you talked of calcium balance and such things. What is it all about?"

I've never been asked the question in just that manner—but that more or less summarizes the questions I get concerning the minerals and elements and the part they play in your good health.

There are two major reasons for including good mineral sources in the diet. In the first place they are important in the structure of the body, making up part of the bones, teeth, muscles and tissue. Secondly, many vital chemical reactions in the body cannot occur unless certain minerals are present. These minerals and elements must come from outside sources.

The most common mineral in the human body is calcium. As you well know, it is an important component of the bones and teeth. But it does other things quite as important. It helps to regulate cardiac contractions. It plays a part in the coagulation

202

of the blood. It activates many of the enzymes which participate in your digestive system. It is an important ingredient in keeping the nervous system in proper function. As well as being found in cheese and milk, calcium also can be obtained from broccoli, kale and mustard greens.

Chlorine, the chief source of which is table salt (sodium chloride), is secreted as hydrochloric acid in the stomach. It maintains the acid-alkali balance of the blood and helps maintain normal cardiac action.

Liver and many vegetables contain cobalt and copper which are required in small quantities to prevent secondary anemia.

Fluorine has been added to the municipal water supply in many communities where the water's normal content is low as it is believed necessary in traces to prevent dental caries, that is, tooth decay.

Iodine regulates the function of the thyroid gland by facilitating the production of thyroxine which participates in the regulation of growth, and the nervous, muscular, circulatory and reproductive systems. A deficiency of iodine will cause simple goiter, cretinism and lowered mental and physical activity. Iodized salt is a principal source and seafood, especially saltwater fish, supplies the element in quantity.

Meats, liver, oysters and soybeans supply the body with iron which is needed for the formation of hemoglobin—the respiratory pigment—of the red blood cells. The ferrous form of many other elements and metals are the most readily absorbed by the human body. A deficiency of iron will cause a secondary anemia.

Magnesium, which you probably know best as the ingredient used in flares, is necessary in minute quantities for the proper functioning of the neuromuscular system and to maintain the normal structure of growing tissue. Cocoa and nuts are principal sources.

Manganese is important for reproduction, lactation and growth. It helps hemoglobin synthesis, is necessary for the storage of vitamin B_1, and prevents the depositing of liver fat. Sources include lettuce and kale.

Potassium, necessary for growth, is also important in muscular contraction, cardiac action and transmission of the nerve impulses. A wide variety of vegetables yield necessary amounts of potassium.

Phosphorus is an essential part of all cells and plays an important role in protein metabolism. It is required for normal tooth and bone structure and is found in many meats and fish.

Sodium, the other ingredient of table salt, regulates water balance in the body and maintains the acid-alkali balance. A deficiency may cause dehydration, nausea, weakness and muscle cramps. Sodium also is found in many seafoods.

Sulphur is an important constituent of many amino acids, hormones, enzymes and vitamins, and a deficiency will affect the functions of all these important substances. Meats and fish are rich in sulphur supply.

Last, but not least, zinc—in trace amounts—is found necessary for normal growth. Seafoods and meats are good sources.

Salt and Water _____

*The first and worst of all frauds
is to cheat one's self.*

P. J. Bailey: FESTUS

BECAUSE IT IS EASIER to give up salt and water than "sweets" many reducing regimes have restricted these two items.

I disagree with this practice!

In following the diet prescribed herein, salt and water should not be restricted. There is no need for it.

Most authorities are agreed now that water retention in a person who is dieting is not permanent and that the failure to lose weight during a diet cannot be attributed to this factor for any length of time.

Many physicians have dehydrated a patient after there has been a failure to lose weight and the patient has insisted that he has strictly observed the diet. These patients usually are only deceiving the physician; in many instances deceiving themselves, too, by utilizing unconscious mechanisms involving rationalizations and repressions.

Attempts at dehydration are fruitless after a few weeks. When a few pounds are lost through the help of salt restriction, mercurial diuretics and ammonium chloride, there is no further

205

loss. What does happen, however, is more serious. In practically all cases the patient develops symptoms due to a lack of sufficient sodium chloride and is forced to retire defeated in the battle against obesity.

It takes only a week or two of normal water intake for the body to regain the few pounds of water lost in dehydration. It is impractical and unwise to expect persons to remain dehydrated —after they have dieted—for the rest of their lives. The idea of dehydration, prevalent in former treatment of obesity, was based mostly on the desire of patients who wished an easier way to attain their goal than by giving up "sweets."

Salt restriction is necessary under certain medical conditions. These are cardiac failure and certain kidney and liver diseases. Often a strict low-sodium regime is imposed on cardiacs to help prevent heart failure. It is silly to expect obese people to live like this unnecessarily.

Table salt and most salts found in various foods are sodium chloride. Sodium keeps water in the tissues. This is a desirable function up to a point. But in certain diseases where the heart is failing as a pump, the normal amount of sodium in the body will keep more water in the tissues than can be handled comfortably and safely. In these cases there may be difficulty in breathing because the lung tissues become waterlogged; the lower limbs may become swollen (popularly called "dropsy"); and the abdomen becomes swollen (ascites).

The restriction of sodium is often a life-saving procedure in cases of cardiac failure because retained water is excreted and the patient can breathe more easily. Edema (the condition of waterlogged tissue) disappears. It is imperative in such cases to keep the patient on a salt-restricted diet all his life, though there has been some controversy recently in the matter of sodium restriction even for cardiacs.

There is no doubt that sodium is necessary in some instances. So the amount of the restriction is important. If the intake is minimal, an undesirable situation can develop due to an imbalance of the sodium-potassium ratio in the body.

But even in cardiac cases it is never necessary to restrict water. Extra water is readily looked after by the kidney. Salt is responsible for water retention, and where salt is restricted, water will not be retained by the tissues.

Sufficient water intake is necessary in order to provide for the various chemical reactions in cells and tissues.

Unless there is medical indication to the contrary, then, salt and water need not be restricted in a diet regime. This is a matter for your physician to decide.

During the weight reduction period, the losses registered on the scale will not only indicate the fat lost from the body, but will also show the shifts in water balance in the body. This can prove a most deceptive and discouraging effect to the sincere dieter.

Extremely obese individuals will usually lose a great amount of weight during the first week of dieting. They find that in subsequent weeks the results of their dieting are not quite as rewarding when they check their scales. The great loss at the beginning of the diet regime is, of course, due mainly to water loss.

A person who is, say, fifty pounds overweight, may lose six to nine pounds in the first week of dieting and then drop down to a three-to-four-pound loss for several weeks; then to two pounds and to one pound in the later weeks. This happens despite the fact that the effort of strict dieting remains unchanged throughout the entire process.

Water lost or retained is unimportant. Eventually there will be an adjustment. The retained water will be excreted later.

It is well to remember this, for I have found that some dieters unaware of this mechanism will decide, after losing a great deal of weight in the first week, that they do not need to diet quite as seriously in the remaining weeks.

How often has a patient reported to me: "Well, I lost eight

207

pounds the first week and therefore I felt I needn't be so strict with myself. By trying half as hard I should be able to lose four pounds a week hereafter."

Unfortunately this thesis doesn't hold true. The great bulk of the lost weight in the first week is merely water. It will require as much effort in the second week to lose four pounds, and as much effort in later weeks to lose two pounds or one pound.

I have seen a person one hundred pounds overweight lose as much as fourteen pounds in the first week of dieting. A person seeking to lose fifteen pounds all told, may lose perhaps four pounds in the same period. Yet each has put the same effort into dieting. The greater the obesity, the more the first week will reward your effort. Later in the regime, the grossly obese person will drop three pounds with as much effort as the moderately obese person does one pound. It is unfair to judge the weight losses comparatively unless on this basis.

Another "disappointing" part of the diet regime is the phenomenon known as the *lag period*. After a patient has been dieting for many weeks and has lost some twenty to thirty pounds, the scale will suddenly show no loss whatsoever for one or two weeks. This in spite of just as strict observance of the diet.

The patient is understandably dismayed. Morale is likely to sink and it becomes more difficult for the patient to make the necessary sacrifices in dieting.

What happens is that fat is being lost during this lag period, but more water is being retained. This water will be excreted at a later date if the dieter persists in his regime.

Ofttimes several pounds of water will be retained by a dieting woman for a week or so due to the menstrual period.

The dilemma facing the physician when a lag period occurs is whether it has been caused by water retention or by the patient's slackening of effort. Naïve patients will lie about their failure to observe their diet strictly. They expect the physician to believe that they have followed the diet to the letter and pull a magic trick from a hat to make up for the lack of loss.

If there only were a trick!

But there isn't, aside from the trick of dieting.

Another instance in which water retention is unjustly blamed is in the case of extremely obese persons whose regular intake of food is so great that a normal person's intake constitutes dieting to them. These people will rationalize their failure at following the prescribed diet by claiming that water retention is preventing them from losing enough weight.

As has been pointed out before, the obese person must eat more than normal in order to give himself enough nourishment to maintain his overweight body. Thus, if such a person starts to eat what he might consume were he of normal weight, he will lose weight. This, to such a person, is considered dieting. More strict diet is "too much of a sacrifice," unless he has been able to attain insight to the underlying reasons of his obesity.

When such a person fails to follow the strict diet prescribed— but does not tell his physician about it and blames the slow results on water retention—the physician can be easily misled.

To understand just what restriction of salt may do to you, you need only recall your own experiences in extremely hot weather. Heat prostration is caused by the body's expelling sodium in perspiration. A common practice in recent years has been to prescribe salt tablets for persons who do heavy work in excess heat or who perspire excessively.

A great deal of sodium is lost in perspiration. Under excessive conditions heat prostration—or so-called sunstroke—may occur. What happens is that the blood pressure falls and many features of shock result. The patient will complain of fatigue, weakness and dizziness. There may also be nausea and vomiting.

Addison's disease, the result of adrenal gland insufficiency, is brought about by the failure of this gland to retain salt in the body. The symptoms are similar to that of heat prostration and are caused by the same mechanism which involves the lack of sodium chloride. Similar symptoms are experienced by many obese persons who have been subjected to a restricted salt regime. They are penalized unnecessarily because salt restriction is of no value in true weight reduction.

Dehydration similarly is of little value on a diet regime.

I have observed in many patients, during a period of temporary water retention, that while the scale will not show a loss of weight, the tape measure will show a loss of fat. Often patients have told me that during a lag period, even though the scale did not reflect loss, they have been able to get into a smaller size dress or pull in another notch on their belts.

Retained water apparently does not affect the body measurements much. Fat, however, does; and all efforts must be directed to fat reduction instead of dehydration.

A rather crude example of the way this water acts is seen in a sponge. A sponge does not bulge when saturated and the body's fat absorbs water in much the same way as the sponge. An athlete will lose several pounds during a contest due to perspiration. This weight will return immediately he drinks sufficient water to quench his thirst. His physical appearance will change none.

If measurements are affected by water retention it will be only in a case of cardiac failure or liver cirrhosis, and only after an extremely large quantity of water has been retained. Where abnormal water retention is noted in an obese individual, a medical assessment should be made so that the reason can be determined. Such individuals are rare and usually have an impaired liver, kidney disease or an unrecognized cardiac failure.

While it may be easier to give up salt than sweets, salt restriction is unnecessary and often unwise. There is even less reason for restricting water.

The only restrictions in a diet should be sweets, starches and fats.

Side Effects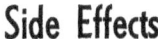

A fat belly does not produce a fine sense.

St. Jerome: DE VIRIS ILLUSTRIBUS

IT IS CHARACTERISTIC that patients on a weight reduction regime will say they feel better than usual.

This sense of well-being often surprises dieters. Folklore has led them to believe that untold miseries would be their lot while dieting. Yet ninety per cent of them find their general health improving.

I have had dieters tell me they are able to accomplish more in every area of life. Some say they can breathe more easily; as the fat melts away there is less pressure against the diaphragm and thorax. Many have admitted to an added sense of self-respect in that their bodies are cleaner and better-looking. Others say they feel a sense of accomplishment in that they have done a major job well.

The remaining ten per cent come up with complaints and symptoms of side effects due to some aspect of their dieting.

Some of the complaints are bizarre and are based on the emotional context of obesity and dieting. Some are incidental and coincidental and not related to dieting and obesity. Some

211

are caused by the medication used to assist in the weight reduction. Some result from the nature of the high-protein diet. Some are caused by the physical and metabolic aspects of dieting involving hypoglycemia, the temporary lowering of the glucose level of the blood.

Let us examine these complaints and see what and how valid they are.

The term "psychosomatic" need not be explained to you. It has become a fairly common word in our vocabulary. You understand that many complaints and symptoms are related to an expression of an emotional need. Physicians' waiting-rooms are full of persons who believe that their symptoms are related to some serious organic illness, but whose symptoms are nothing more than an unconscious protest against an intolerable life situation; or a means of escape; or an attention-getting device; or a secondary gain.

These unfortunate individuals are only conscious that they suffer with real pain, or are afflicted with a real symptom. Their afflictions are not imaginary. They are truly experienced and suffered, but the underlying dynamics is in the emotional sphere and results from some repression or other. Pain may be caused by an injury or an organic disease. But it may also be experienced as a stimulus from the higher cerebral centers in the nervous system because of an emotional need for self-punishment owing to a feeling of guilt.

Some of the psychodynamics of obesity have been covered earlier in this book. Many persons, to whom obesity has served a neurotic need, will escape into another symptom when the escape into overeating can no longer be utilized. These patients tell of many bizarre symptoms and cause the physician much harassment during a weight reduction regime.

Upon questioning, it will be discovered that many patients have had the newly complained of symptoms before they started dieting. But these symptoms have become more pronounced and troublesome since the diet regime was undertaken. In most cases discussion and the allaying of fear is all that is needed to solve the new problem. In others major depth analysis or psychoanalysis becomes obviously imperative if the reducing program is to be concluded successfully.

Some patients will complain of a "lump in the throat," known in the medical profession as globus hystericus. Some feel a pressure on the chest, or tension headaches, or migraine headaches. Some complain of tremors, or "peculiar sensations" under the skin (paresthesia). Others will "escape" into sleep and complain of fatigue and constant sleepiness. A syndrome known as the "anxiety attack" is complained about on rare occasions, taking the form of rapid beating of the heart, profuse perspiration, a nameless fear and a feeling of impending doom.

Many fears and tensions which have been crudely cloaked by the fortress of fat will push closer to the consciousness during a weight reduction regime. Anxiety attacks are the result. Practically all the patients have had similar attacks previously, but they become more noticeable during dieting.

Despite all these symptoms, complaints and side effects, it is to the benefit of the patient that they are out in the open. As recognizable complaints there is at least a chance of handling them in a mature manner.

Symptoms such as nervousness and increased irritability are caused by the denial of the escape into overeating. Persons who have been accustomed to eating gluttonously as their answer to problems will at times, during dieting, be troubled by bad temper in expressing unconscious hostility to someone they are required to love.

Many obese persons resent either unconsciously or consciously the need to make sacrifices in order to lose weight. Gourmandizing has become a way of life for them. They are all too eager to find some excuse which they can use as a rationalization in order not to undergo the rigors of dieting. Any incidental illness not related in any way to their dieting will be utilized by them for this purpose.

During any epidemic of upper respiratory diseases, which are most common in winter, some dieters feel that their reduced intake has "weakened" them in some fashion so that they fall easy prey to the infection.

One housewife, who was on a weight reduction regime with me when her husband contracted a virus infection during such an epidemic, nursed him for more than a week. Her two children then ran fevers during the following week. When, after her family recovered, she succumbed, she was convinced that it was dieting which had weakened her and was the principal cause of her illness.

How she reasoned this is almost inconceivable as no other member of her family had been dieting and she had almost exhausted herself in caring for them before she herself succumbed to the virus infection.

Of course, folklore has contributed greatly to this attitude. Allergies, skin rashes and toothaches are but a few of the afflictions which have been attributed to dieting.

Let us not deny that there are some complaints which can be attributed to some physical aspects of dieting. Medication used as an adjunct in dieting may have side effects and these were discussed in the chapter on "Medication."

Drying of the mouth may be caused by the amphetamine family of hunger-curbers and this is enhanced when atropine is added.

The most side effects noted are caused by the multicolored tablets which contain thyroid and other drug mixtures. These, it was pointed out previously, are not to be utilized.

The use of phenobarbital or other sedatives, to counteract the overstimulation of amphetamine in sensitive individuals, may in turn oversedate the patient.

Bulk laxatives may cause an undesirable feeling of overdistension or bloating in some patients.

Ill-advised persons who self-medicate may have symptoms referable to overdosage.

Faddist diets involving serious omissions of high-quality foods may cause symptoms related to some vitamin or mineral lack.

Constipation, varying in severity, may occur to individuals who have been accustomed to a rich diet for many years and are then put on a high-protein weight reduction diet. This constipation may be increased if water is unnecessarily limited in addition. Such patients have been found to have always had a constipation problem, but the degree has been increased in the diet regime. The intestinal tract in these patients sometimes lacks sufficient muscle tone. The change of diet from one rich in carbohydrates and fats to one in which these classes of foods are curtailed may be constipating.

This is not a serious problem and does not generally persist. It may be necessary to use a saline purgative or bulk laxative for a varying period whenever necessary.

The gall bladder and liver also are involved to some respect in obesity and in dieting.

Medical students are taught that gall-bladder patients usually are females "fair, fat and forty." These patients complain of nausea, belching, occasional vomiting and pain in the upper right part of the abdomen. They may also have gall-bladder attacks while on a weight losing diet. The attacks are *less frequent than those of normal gall-bladder illness,* as the weight reduction diet generally is similar to that advocated for gall-bladder patients and so serves a sort of double function.

Liver damage is present in most obese persons. In some it is slight while in other cases it can be quite extensive. Autopsies performed on obese persons who have perished due to varying illnesses have revealed that their livers have been infiltrated with fat and were impaired for this reason.

Fatty liver is the early stage of liver disease before cirrhosis sets in. Individuals who diet to lose weight must live off their stored fat. As the liver is the organ which performs the function of converting fat into glucose in metabolism (as described earlier), an impaired liver will not perform the function efficiently. This malfunctioning, of course, will result in some symptoms. The liver will be restored to greater efficiency when the fat stored in that organ is reduced along with the body's fat during dieting.

Faddist diets may start a train of symptoms known as hypoglycemia, a lack of sufficient sugar in the blood. This is a result of what actually amounts to starvation. The common symptoms are dizzy spells, drowsiness, black-outs and periods of feeling faint. These occurrences usually are minimal and not particularly harmful. Harm can come to a person who is not truly overweight but who, in trying to drop several pounds, does not seek a doctor's advice and goes on a starvation diet.

As long as vitamin, mineral and protein needs are supplied to the obese person on a diet, no harm can come of the diet regime. It is not possible for these people to have hypoglycemia following the diet prescribed herein. The large quantity of protein advocated will not create a lowering of the blood's sugar content.

Practically all obese persons who claim to have objectionable symptoms while on a diet generally are utilizing a different escape mechanism when the escape into overeating is denied them. Many naïve patients who have not been properly oriented will interpret such symptoms as evidence that dieting is unhealthy because they need little or no excuse to stop dieting.

Do not be misled by these symptoms; rather be encouraged by them. They mean that your dieting is successful and you should continue. If a halt is called in the dieting, then a stoppage will occur in the weight reduction.

Loss of weight is a grim necessity before obesity results in irreparable damage to the liver.

Psychotherapy

Men look no further than their outsides.

Sir Thomas Browne: RELIGIO MEDICI

"IF OVERWEIGHT IS THE RESULT of overeating, why can't I successfully reduce by dieting?"

That is a question I fully expect to hear. But the answer is obvious. Throughout the book I have attempted to show that persons who have tried to diet on their own have failed to lose weight in most cases.

Earlier chapters have shown conclusively that the patient must have some understanding of the reasons for his overeating before he can start dieting successfully. Under the general heading of understanding of the problem comes the task of psychotherapy.

The difference between success and failure in the treatment of obesity is psychotherapy.

In explaining this to a patient one day the following conversation ensued:

"Just what is psychotherapy? Does it involve lengthy analysis? And does it mean that to lose weight I must spend years in working out my emotional problems by means of analysis?"

217

"The only answer I can give to this over-all question," I replied, "is 'Not necessarily.'

"Most patients fail to realize that any form of guidance given by a medical practitioner, a psychiatrist, analyst, spiritual leader, teacher, social worker, or even friend or parent, is in a sense psychotherapy.

"We call it *supportive psychotherapy*. It attempts to improve the patient's personality and provide emotional support to enhance the patient's sense of security."

The bulk of the psychotherapy given to the obese patient by the practitioner is supportive therapy. Its purpose is to give the patient the opportunity to understand intellectually, at least, the drives that motivate overeating.

Mere knowledge of diets, of calories, and of types of foods, as has been pointed out before, is not sufficient to enable an obese person to reduce to normal weight and to hold at that desirable level.

This supportive, or superficial, psychotherapy is aimed at practical—though necessarily limited—goals. The efforts of the therapist—in this case the physician—are directed at relieving symptoms as they crop up in the conscious realization, to help maintain the patient's self-respect and to increase his sense of security.

In supportive psychotherapy, which physicians utilize not only in treating obesity but other illnesses as well, no attempt is made to get to the root of the illness. Such a process involves major psychoanalysis.

The physician, by listening to his patient's difficulties with understanding and without condemnation, is practicing psychotherapy. Merely allowing the patient to air his difficulties is sufficient to create a greater sense of security in the sufferer. This airing, or ventilation, is known as mental catharsis—cleaning out of the emotional processes. Such therapy is not limited to the doctor-patient relationship. It has been a feature of many religions for centuries; it is a feature of social work, of teaching, and of many professions in which there is a person-to-person contact.

The patient whose obesity is persistent and does not respond to the doctor's supportive psychotherapy will require psychoanalysis or major psychotherapy before a cure is to be hoped for.

The average obesity patient is motivated in seeking a cure by reasons of vanity or health in most cases. Few are aware, or even concerned, with the emotional difficulties behind the overweight. So it is necessary that the patient be educated as to the emotional and neurotic basis of obesity, which is the first block against appropriate treatment.

Even to patients aware of the problem, the expense, time and emotional discomfort involved in major psychotherapy is formidable. Fortunately most obese individuals do not require psychoanalysis, unless one subscribes to the theory that, as all humans have neurotic traits of some sort, all should undergo analysis. This is a ridiculous assumption and reduces human effort almost to training a portion of humanity so that they can analyze the balance of humanity. It cannot be denied that there are many persons who have difficulties and who therefore are personally unhappy and limited in productive usefulness. For these, psychoanalysis is rewarding. They acquire greater personal happiness and become more useful members of society.

No better example can be given than that of the playwright who stagnated for years before undergoing psychoanalysis. Since then, his name has become a household word and his work bids to live long in the history of the theater.

The question of who should be analyzed and who should not is pertinent. Generally the candidate for analysis should be young enough so that the patterns of life are not too set and are therefore capable of investigation. In the case of older people, it is often felt that the life expectancy of the patient is not long enough to have the treatment be of value, considering the length of time analysis may require. It has proved tragic in some cases

219

of older persons who have undergone analysis only to discover that they have chosen the wrong career or are married—out of a neurotic necessity—to a mate who merely fitted into the unhealthy pattern of the neurosis.

For the obese patient to require analysis means only that the patient has not responded to the physician's supportive therapy and other medical measures. Such patients, it has been found, usually have other neurotic traits associated with their obesity. These may be alcoholism or character psychoneurosis in which the person is unable to adjust to such social institutions as marriage, law, or even work.

The obese person should never be persuaded to undergo psychoanalysis. The patient alone should be the best judge of such a necessity after a calm discussion of the various factors pertinent to his particular case.

Most patients have blocks, or objections, to such deep treatment. They are unwilling to surrender the defenses which they have carefully built up around their feelings of inadequacy, their primitive and socially unacceptable longings and their various guilts. I have observed that the only individuals who consent to analysis are those whose unhappinesses have led them desperately to seek help.

It should be obvious, too, that persons of low-normal intelligence are not fit subjects for analysis. Analysis is a process which is difficult even for persons of superior intelligence. Thus it becomes almost an impossible thing for the other type. It might be likened to the equivalent of explaining to an Australian bush native the scientific workings of radio, only to have the listener then reduce it to terms of magic and mysticism.

In the strictest sense of the word, psychotherapy is treatment for the emotional illness at the basis of obesity—or any neurotic symptom—which involves helping the patient adjust to the problem or problems in a more mature manner. Psychotherapy may involve analysis during which the patient's experiences in childhood are explored and examined. This is a process long and tedious. It is necessarily painful in an emotional sense, as well as being expensive. But it does offer the best possibilities of permanent cure.

Often patients unable to diet successfully will undergo psychoanalysis and then resume their treatments for obesity. These stubborn cases find themselves responding much more rapidly to a reducing program once they have gone some way along in analysis.

One such case that comes to mind is that of an industrial research chemist whom we shall call William. He was twenty-eight years old when he came to me weighing 245 pounds.

William is a brilliant man in his field and had earned a Ph.D. at the age of twenty-two. He is the only child of a university professor of English—who died three years before William came to me for treatment. His mother capably took over direction of a small, exclusive private school after the death of her husband.

"My father was a gentle, introverted, impractical and scholarly man," William told me in our talks. "But he was overwhelmed by my mother."

William's description of his mother was "handsome and opulent with a forceful, extroverted and direct personality." The man's love for his father was obviously veiled with contempt for the "henpecking" he allowed, and his love for his mother was colored by fear of her domination.

Aside from the problem of his overweight, William was burdened by other troubles. He was a periodic alcoholic—his drinking linked to every personal crisis he encountered. His undoubted brilliance in his work was the only reason that he was able to obtain and hold various positions. He suffered violent migraine headaches which often lasted as long as three days and occurred at least once a month.

He admitted the reason he wanted to take what he called "extra pounds" off his five-foot-eight frame "is a girl." William

221

had never been married and his social life, in his own words, "was meager." He had never formed anything resembling a permanent attachment with any of his female friends.

Despite his overweight he was not unattractive but was quite conscious of his feeling of inadequacy with the opposite sex.

"There's no one to blame but myself for my failure with women," he had said. "But now that I have met this girl, who works at the plant I do, I have developed a strong desire to reach a more normal weight."

Ordinary measures were only of limited success in his case. He lost twenty-two pounds and was unable to go beyond that. He blamed himself.

"I plain and simple lack will power. For instance, I get overwhelming desires to eat all sorts of sweet things or delicacies before I go to bed.

"When I try to diet, my migraine bothers me much more. It seems to me that there must undoubtedly be some sort of psychosomatic relationship between my attacks of migraine, my obesity and my drinking."

William himself suggested that he might be helped by psychoanalysis. After a year of therapy he resumed his obesity treatment. This time his success was complete. He dropped to 185 pounds within a few months and lost another twenty pounds later.

He told me that analysis led him to the discovery that he was attempting to ape his mother in almost all things during his life.

"This mimicry obviously led me to become overweight so that I could approach the female configuration of my mother. It seems that unconscious contempt for my father's weakness and my respect, tinged with fear, for my mother's strength, directed me to imitate her."

At this writing, William had started his third year of analysis. His obesity state no longer existed and his migraine attacks had all but disappeared. His alcoholism and inability to love had been somewhat rectified, but still required extensive therapy. But he claimed the most happiness out of having come down to 156 pounds. This he did in stages so that he could absorb loose skin after each session.

The importance of psychotherapy in the treatment of obesity has become so recognized that the United States Public Health Service conducted experiments in Boston recently. Part of the results of these experiments were discussed in an earlier chapter. The experiments were attempted to see if treatment from "group therapy"—obese people getting together to discuss their problems among themselves—would be of value. The results were limited, unfortunately, but they did prove again the need for psychotherapy in the treatment of obesity.

The idea of group therapy was tried because therapy involving only individuals cannot be a practical answer to the great bulk of obese patients. This is mainly because of the lack of trained personnel for this work.

However the group therapy idea offers limited results because it requires skillful and well-trained psychiatrists to conduct the groups. In individual analysis, the patient and analyst have a simpler road to traverse in reaching their goal. In group therapy the analyst is faced with a group of persons, each with different likes and dislikes. This cross-current of opinions—and quite possibly some opinions involving the analyst—makes a far more complicated situation to unravel.

The idea of group therapy has blossomed into such organizations as "Fatties Anonymous" which have sprung up in various parts of the United States. These groups invite psychiatrists, physicians and psychologists to address their meetings on the various aspects of obesity, and follow these talks with group discussion. Some individuals have been helped by these methods, but for the greater part these organizations have become a means by which true treatment is evaded and the overweight member's conscience is salved by halfhearted attempts.

One patient of mine who had belonged to a "Fatties Anonymous" club said in paraphrase of Mark Twain's famous remark about the weather:

"They all talk about obesity, but no one really does anything about it."

Before undertaking analysis the patient should have a general discussion of his problems with his physician to see if analysis is advisable. The physician will refer the patient to an analyst—if this is decided upon—and the analyst will in turn direct the patient first to a clinical psychologist for intelligence and personality evaluation through various tests.

Psychoanalysis may require three to five visits to the analyst weekly, each of at least one hour's duration, and the analysis may take anywhere from eighteen months to five years. The results do not involve the creation of a godlike individual, but more of a person whose basic personality remains unchanged to friends, relatives and business associates. What changes do take place will be those of a more calm and reasonable attitude to life's various phases, an increased capacity for the enjoyment of life, a more productive output in the patient's life's work, and a more mature attitude to such things as marriage, children, parents, employer or employees, and society in general.

What does take place in analysis?

First a complete personality study is made of the patient and as complete as possible a life history is recorded. The patient's life is then reconstructed step by step in order to reproduce the origin and development of his obesity—and other neurotic traits.

Then there follows a series of discussions between the patient and the physician about the patient's complaints and problems. These discussions may apparently involve topics not closely connected with the patient's illness. But every topic is related. The therapist will guide the patient's interviews into regions which will give information on the nature of the patient's difficulties. The questions asked are for the purpose of enabling the patient to see for himself the way he reacts to his own experiences.

The patient's understanding is never obtained by being told an opinion of his difficulties. It is, rather, obtained by gaining insight through gradual steps by means of discussions and questions.

Situations which are painful or tend to lessen the patient's self-respect will be repressed, blocked and forgotten. Repressed experiences can only emerge through gradual steps by the patient under the skillful direction of the psychotherapist. It is assumed that the intelligent patient, through discussion, will be able to analyze the factors underlying his difficulties and be able to make the necessary changes.

Importance is placed on the study of unconscious situations which involve unpleasantness to the patient and have therefore been repressed. An attempt is made to bring to the patient's awareness the unconscious motivations which have been disturbing his life.

The analyst is careful not to suggest interpretations of the patient's symbols. The patient must discover for himself the meanings of the products which emerge from his unconscious.

The analyst utilizes the process of transference—in which the patient assumes the same emotional attitude to the analyst which he previously held toward an individual, usually a parent, who played an important role in his life—to call the patient's attention to the irrationalities of his behavior. It is thus that the patient becomes aware of many of the memories leading back as far as childhood and so discovers the source of his neurosis.

Weight Watching —————————————————

To lengthen thy life, lessen thy meals.

Benjamin Franklin: POOR RICHARD'S ALMANAC

IF YOU HAVE NOW REACHED the point where your weight should be about normal, you will have done a creditable job.

But, while having won a major victory, you will still face a long period of "cold war." You will have to maintain your level, and thus will have joined the ranks of the "weight watchers."

The intensity and length of your weight-watching battle depends solely upon your reason for losing excess weight. Some persons are strongly motivated by the temporary advantage that being of normal weight will bring them. For example:

Young men and women will lose their excess fat during a period of courting. They will overcome their strong orality temporarily in order to win a sweetheart.

A woman who feels she is losing her husband to some "charmer" will be strongly motivated to regain her slimness.

A man who has been told by his physician that his years are numbered because of his obesity may effectively lose weight.

But when these persons feel that the danger has passed, or that they have attained the object which weight reduction was to bring for them, their unconscious drives and demands for excessive food will be reasserted and they will regain the excess fat.

Another factor to be watchful of is that of "self reward." A good many obese people have utilized the habit of eating as a reward mechanism. When they attain normal weight, their sense of accomplishment is accountably great. They will have received compliments from friends and relatives and will be regarded with added respect due to their improved appearance.

As they know of only one way of rewarding themselves and feel they must be rewarded for their accomplishment, they will go on an eating binge. The sense of this is no different than that of an alcoholic who has successfully abstained for a long period and celebrates his accomplishment with a few drinks. The hard earned profits are quickly lost.

To achieve a permanent victory over obesity you must first have some degree of insight or understanding of the mechanism underlying your excessive demands for food. As has been pointed out, some persons will find only a superficial intellectual insight adequate in controlling their obesity. A few, however, require emotional insight, and major psychoanalysis is involved.

A number of the case studies presented in this book have shown the need for psychotherapy. The majority of obese persons, however, do not need this emotional insight. For them the superficial intellectual insight of their problem is sufficient and they can gain this insight by cooperating with their physicians.

Individuals are prone to obesity during five critical periods of life. These are times when they are likely to feel most insecure and their oral demands for food, therefore, become excessive.

These Five Ages of Fat are:

Puberty, when the pressure of adult life is imminent.

Marriage, when an important adjustment to a new way of living must be made.

Pregnancy, when responsibility for a new helpless individual must be assumed—and fathers-to-be are just as prone to this critical time as the prospective mothers.

Menopause, when the realization is made that youth has departed.

Old Age, when worry develops over chronic illnesses and the impending dissolution of the personality.

No matter with how much ease or difficulty you have achieved your normal weight in the treatment, you now must constantly watch your weight for many months, or even years.

You realize now that the basic difference between thin people, people of normal weight, and obese people is the amount of food intake and the unconscious control of this intake which permits the normal-weight people to maintain that normality unconsciously.

Obese people will not be satisfied with the amount of food involved in normal eating, feeling that it is quite inadequate. Thin or normal-weight persons may overeat while in the presence of others as an attention-gaining device, but they eat sufficiently little when alone to make up for this overindulgence. Obese persons will at all times overeat or eat frequent meals interspersed with snacks.

To stay at any specified weight, every individual must eat approximately the same amount.

As has been fully described, the course of weight reduction will involve large losses on the scale during the first few weeks. These weight losses include large quantities of water. In later weeks less and less weight will be lost as reflected on the scale; but the tape measure will show the results of the dieting.

Conversely, after achieving normal weight, a person can put on excess weight again by overeating at about the same rate as it came off. As much as seven pounds can go on in one week, and successive weeks will see four, then three, then two pounds added until sufficient weight is gained to balance the amount of food consumed. The top limit is reached when the extra fat, which also needs nourishment, will exactly balance the amount of extra food intake.

An obese individual who rewards himself with a series of big dinners after the deprivation of a diet regime may discover to his consternation that he has regained many pounds after a week of celebration. Such a discovery may easily destroy the morale of the weight watcher, especially if he becomes convinced that the struggle against overweight is futile.

Any number of pounds gained in one week of overindulgence after achieving normal weight can be removed in a short period of returning to the strict diet of the regime.

For many persons it may be necessary to forego the sensual pleasures of eating rich desserts and foods almost permanently. This is so that they may indulge in more bulk of other foods and still hold the line of normal weight.

Weight watching is doing *consciously* what people of normal weight do *unconsciously*.

The first step in watching your weight is knowing your exact weight status periodically. This is done by weighing yourself *once a week* on the *same scale* at the *same time* of day wearing the *same amount of clothes*. This will bring about the most exact correlation possible.

Weighing yourself more often than once a week will make you "scale happy." Under such circumstances, your exact weight status will never be known. There are many shifts in water balance in the body, such as during a woman's menstrual period or a man's excessive perspiration, and these will be reflected in a daily see-saw on the scale.

A patient who has overindulged in food one day may gain a false sense of security the next should he step on the scale and find that he has not gained any weight, or has perhaps even lost a pound. This may encourage further excessive eating and within a week, to the weight watcher's dismay, many pounds will have been added.

Some persons may find that after watching their food intake carefully over a period of weeks, their weight has increased a few pounds. This is caused by temporarily retained water; but it can be a discouraging thing to discover.

By checking once a week, under the conditions outlined above, a better picture of your weight watching is achieved. You should carefully record your weight each week. If a pound or two is added, you must "go into training" immediately to remove this so that a more serious return to a diet regime is not necessary later.

It is possible that after achieving your normal weight, you will continue to lose weight. This is due usually to an overstrict diet regime after the normal weight has been accomplished. Your weight watching will prevent further weight loss, for in these circumstances you will be encouraged to eat more to hold your weight at the desired level.

The first weeks of weight watching will indicate to you just what and how much food is necessary to maintain your normal weight. You may find that you must omit sweets, or snacks, or rich desserts permanently. You may find that restriction of food every second, or third, or fourth week is necessary. Best of all, you may find that you have permanently overcome your excessive desires for food and will unconsciously be able to maintain your normal weight within a short time of having completed your diet regime.

Every dieter who achieves a weight reduction to the proper level will discover what his normal level is early in the weight-watching period. This should be checked with your physician. Many authorities have endeavored to list the most desirable weight for men and women for particular height, build and age. But the factors of individual and familial differences are difficult ones for the layman to include in that calculation. For that reason your physician is the person best able to determine what your normal weight should be.

It should be apparent to you now that you should not attempt to start or continue a weight-reduction program without your physician's help.

First he is needed to help you understand why you are obese—what your particular reason is for the obesity neurosis you have developed. Then with his help you can set about losing weight. He will prescribe a diet fitted to your needs, he will administer hunger-curbing medication should you require it, he will determine if you need vitamin supplements, and, most important, he will help you to pass through any of the trying periods you may encounter.

An important thing for each person who has successfully lost many pounds to do is to have the physician set a top level of weight for future days. This level is never to be exceeded. The knowledge acquired during the diet regime should be utilized in keeping the balance and reducing from this top level if it is reached. If at any time the patient goes over the top level, he should return for treatment.

Some persons will have one relapse, others may have two, and some may even experience three relapses. But any person who has held at normal—or within the top level figure—for two or three years, is likely to hold that way for the rest of his life.

The problem must never get out of hand. If you start to regain weight, cannot successfully cut back within the next few weeks, and go over the top level, *do not wait* until you have regained all your weight before returning to your physician for treatment. This will only involve a vicious seesaw of excessive obesity to normal to excess ad infinitum. It is not a solution to the problem of obesity.

The person who has attained insight, lost excessive weight through dieting and then carefully watched weight, will find that the problem of remaining at normal weight becomes less and less difficult as time goes on. Soon the process becomes a conditioned reflex and will be quite "painless."

231

Before you know it, you will have acquired the unconscious "governor" of those persons who never have had difficulty in staying at a normal weight.

When that day comes you will have successfully conquered your number one health enemy.

Index